WELL AFTER WAR

James M. McGarrity

To Senator Sherrod Brown
Thank you for your
commitment to veterans.
with regards & respect
James M. McGarrity
Dec 2011

2011
Revised and Edited by
James M. McGarrity
Based on his 2009 memoir:
CHECKPOINT ONE FOUR:
Printing by
FedEx Office, Branch 1229
3757 W. Market St
Fairlawn, OH 44333

TO MY WIFE: DOROTHY
MY CHILDREN: KELLY AND MICHAEL
MY SISTER: DIANE
Our Mother,
MARIAN BLINN MCGARRITY
(1927-1977)

PTSD

SHELL-SHOCKED WW I

BATTLE FATIGUE WW II

VIETNAM SYNDROME: VN

PREFACE

This is the story of my day-to-day journey, forty years after Vietnam, and how I dealt with the complex realities, yet primal simplicities of Posttraumatic Stress Disorder (PTSD).

During my first four years of therapy, I watched fellow veterans struggle with even the most basic expressions to describe their emotional pains. I imagined how a detailed record might someday encourage veterans down the same road I had traveled, where even-though distant and commonly frightening, I believed a better life was possible.

Further-on in my journey, as I became an advocate and mentor for veterans of all generations, I saw how my story might also be a resource for family members; clergy, and especially: social workers and mental health clinicians as I detailed my first years of dialogue with VA mental health providers.

These remarkable and devoted people of the Veterans Administration helped me realize why I became the person I was: Not only a Marine veteran of the Vietnam War, but the child who carried his harsh experiences into the military, predisposing me as most clinicians believe, to be especially vulnerable to the long term effects of trauma, even as others might be affected less — or some far worse — or perhaps, some not at all.

It took some doing, but therapy helped me realize why for nearly four decades, I responded to the world in a different, more frightening and unpredictable way than those around me.

I began to see why abusing drugs, and fighting, and testing the limits of self-destruction were part of a complex need within me to override the persistent memories of a day at a small bridge into anything that might relieve the guilt; the shattered self esteem; the distrust of authority and a hypersensitive need for safety.

If these things sound familiar, or if you know someone who has been traumatized, I believe my story will help you find your way or point the way for others.

INTRODUCTION

Tens of thousands of every age, gender, culture and military branch, have been diagnosed as I, with PTSD: Posttraumatic Stress Disorder — a mental condition so distinctly life-altering, that at times we can appear as if being stamped from the same mold.

But when struck with trauma, our individual fears can hinge the past with the present, purging emotions locked in our memories during moments of great fear: like the smell of a drunken parent at your bedside, or the gut-wrenching cries of your mother, trying her best to fend-off an abusive partner.

From these moments on, those memories of fear became locked in our unconscious, affecting how we would relate to the world each-day-after. Including the memories of our most terrifying moments — our military traumas.

One of these memory-storing organs is the hippocampus. It lies deep within the center of our brain and resembles a ram's curved horns. Its job is to stores facts, like: remembering directions or that every Tuesday our Group meets or, what it felt like to burn our leg on a motorcycle exhaust 20 years ago.

This ability to store facts, especially facts about what hurt, danger and fear means to us personally, makes the hippocampus a powerful force in our daily lives; sending out signals of chemically-charged hormones when danger seems eminent, energizing our hearts and lungs and muscles to respond, based on the **logic** the hippocampus has recorded during our life-lessons of what danger means.

Facing danger based on facts and logic works fairly well for us modern humans, as throughout history we became more intelligent and moral and avoiding of violent conflict through resolution.

But for our ancient ancestors to survive in a world of split-second danger and death, violent and immediate reactions were necessary. Because of that need, early human brains were locked-and-loaded for instant action, poised to respond in our most primal and aggressive manner.

Known as the amygdala; sometimes referred to as "the lizard;" our amygdalae don't care one bit about facts. Its only concern is our survival at the moment.

The lizard's power lies in its dark warehouse of fearful emotional memories, where one of three ancient survival actions will be energized: fight, flight or freeze.

These primitive reactions caused our cave-dwelling ancestors to strike at the mere sound of a twig snapping in the darkness; a sound their amygdalae had recorded throughout their upbringing as only one thing — survival at any cost!

But as the human brain evolved, the logically-disposed hippocampus grew and attained power over the lizard, cementing its ability to restrain its cranial companion's hypersensitive responses like a throttle controls an engine.

This "throttle effect" prompted humans to respond to danger in more dispassionate ways and use its powerful old cohort the amygdala like a force in reserve instead of "on point."

But what happens when the modern brain becomes overwhelmed? Like for example when extreme horror occurs and the lizard, who is always there, observing, examining danger based on our "old fears," erupts; called to action; choking-back the hippocampus and flooding the brain with its toxic stew of reactionary hormones?

According to experts the result can be a "burned-in" recollection of a traumatic event as the hippocampus becomes saturated and parts of it "drowns;" replacing memories based on logic with newly captured memories of horror and death; abandonment and guilt; fear of insanity and the helplessness of betrayal.

This is where forever after, those of us with PTSD will act irrationally during moments in which our brains can only recognize a fight or flight, do or die situation: Like preparing to kill or be killed at the sound of a twig snapping in the darkness.

This is what happened to me on an October morning in 1967 when our convoy was ambushed on a desolate stretch of highway in South Vietnam.

What happened that morning was burned into my being.

This is that story.

I

A LONG WAY FROM HOME

We were going!

The day most of us had hoped for since arriving at radio school had finally arrived:

We were going to Vietnam!

It was January, 1967. Nearly ten months had passed since I graduated from the Marine Corps Recruit Depot at Parris Island, South Carolina, followed with several weeks of weapons and tactics instruction at the Corps,' Infantry Training Regiment at Camp Geiger — located somewhere in the endless boondocks and Copperhead-infested-swamps abutting Camp Lejeune, North Carolina.

Following training at Geiger we received the standard thirty days of leave before reporting to our individual training assignments. I went to the Marine base at San

Diego, California where for twenty-six weeks myself and seventy-or-so fellow Marines from around the country, would learn to operate a variety of field radios including an intense course in Morse code. The result was what some considered the best communicators in the Corps at the time and even though Morse code (CW: constant wave) was phased-out by the 1970's, its value to frustrate enemy operatives caused it to be reintroduced into Marine special operations command units (MARSOC) in later conflicts.

My best friend at radio school was a native Californian — Phil Jones. He was raised, and his parents still lived in an upscale suburb of Los Angeles — maybe Azusa.

Following graduation we received a 30 day leave en lieu of reporting to Camp Pendleton, California for advanced training prior to our 13 month tours in Vietnam. I arranged (I would have lied if I had to) to spend the night before check-in at Phil's family home.

It was an elaborately arranged rendezvous, that if pressed to justify I'd swear was nothing more than two friends meeting-up to march off to war.

In truth, my anxiety over the uncertainties of finding my way to the base on my own and possibly being late to check-in and so-on and so-on had overwhelmed me.

Even with the details of meeting Phil in Los Angeles worked-out by expensive, long distance phone calls from my mother's home in Akron, my stomach was in knots the morning we prepared to drive to Hopkins Airport in Cleveland, Ohio.

Prone to her own bouts of anxiety, my mother had a deep-seeded relationship with fear of the unknown, and throughout her years of mental instability, especially after her second marriage, she had become increasingly dependent on prescription drugs to quell their most frightening symptoms.

Ever mindful of signs of worry, the morning of my departure, she rummaged through her stash of pills for the perfect tranquilizer. Her second husband, my stepfather; who by the way never sought nor earned the title, was a pharmacist. It goes without saying that our kitchen cupboard was loaded with a stockpile of powerful medications: A fact common for the times.

For like many urban neighborhoods in the 1960's, especially "Old World" European ones, a private; some might say sinister relationship existed among its businessmen; the church; the law; the mob and local bigwigs. Foremost within these microcosms of life, the engine driving commerce, aside from the forests of smokestacks, was a one block or two strip of every merchant that most families required. Anchoring the tidy storefronts, bars and bakeries was the ubiquitous corner drug store, with the second floor interminably a doctor's or dentist's office.

This close-knit club of professionals enjoyed and profited from their cozy relationships. As upstairs, the doctors wrote the prescriptions — and downstairs his crony filled them.

It was the perfect arrangement! As the respected medical men and civil-minded benefactors on multiple levels understood, they would never be accused of wrongdoings. And so, a wink and a nod was all that was needed to control not only their own wives, but the wives of neighborhood pals:

What could it hurt, they would have asked themselves? You feed "the little woman" 'speed' to get the kids off to school and the house cleaned. And later, after returning home from work and dinner was done and the brats tucked-in for the night, the 'downers' she'd been given to "come down" should kick-in leaving her "knocked out" on the sofa.

It was shortly after her marriage that this became my mother's world.

But trying to balance powerful drugs of opposing synergy can have frightening results. I must say, that during my teenage years, I did find it unusual that many nights, after the TV channels and the hangouts had shut down, I'd find her on her knees, scrubbing the kitchen floor as if she could see the germs.

Some might ask why I didn't think her behavior was unusual. All I can say is: It was just the way life was at our house. So when she handed me the two capsules the morning I was leaving for Vietnam — I swallowed them!

No big deal.

Sure — no big deal. Except that by the time we arrived at Cleveland Hopkins Airport I could barely keep my eyes open, and since we were running late due to a wrong turn, my mother dropped me at the entrance and sped-off to find a parking place.

As she disappeared into a world of colorless and salt-stained cars, I wandered through the terminal to the gate and directly onto the tarmac. My canvas sea bag was slung like a giant green sausage over one shoulder as I followed other shivering passengers single file toward the mobile stairway and relief from the biting Lake Erie wind.

I guess I was so out-of-it mentally that I didn't give much thought to the fact that I might never see my mother again. But once inside, I plopped myself matter-of-factly into a seat by a window.

Through the frost blotted porthole I could see the ground crew preparing to tow the platform back to the terminal. The last passengers aboard were stowing their jackets in carryon compartments as others fumbled with their seat belts, settling-in and fiddling with the waft of tiny ventilators above them. The whirr of turbines countered the din of human activity until little was heard but the repetitive ebb of mechanical reverberation. Then suddenly the engines idled-down and the interior became quite quiet. The pilot's voice resonated throughout the compartment and passengers paused.

"Ladies and gentlemen," the pilot said. "I have received a request by a mother whose son has just boarded the plane and is leaving for Vietnam. Please be patient as we will only be delayed for a few minutes."

The ground crew nudged the platform tight against the fuselage and air rushed through the compartment as a stewardess unsealed the hatch.

The fact that it was me: the "son going to Vietnam" he mentioned, didn't register. Then I saw an attractive woman with jet black hair coming down the aisle, scanning the rows of seats from one side to the other. It was my mother. When she spotted me she leaned across the passenger beside me in the aisle-seat and hugged me and kissed me and said I love you.

And then she disappeared, almost as quickly as she had arrived. And once again, I fell into a deep sleep.

It was always the craziest thing — flying to California. It was a four hour flight from Cleveland, but with the time difference you arrive about an hour after you leave. So around 11:30 AM, Pacific Time, I was standing in front of LAX. The sun was shining and I was praying that Phil hadn't forgotten my arrival when a car pulled up to the curb and a tall, fatherly looking gentleman exited and walked toward me.

"Are you Jim," Phil's dad said, extending his hand.

I was so glad to see him.

"Yes sir," I answered.

"I expected you to be about eight feet tall," he said, "given the way Phil has talked about you."

I didn't know what to say — I guess I was a little embarrassed

But I had done it! I had reached California and left the gut wrenching anxiety of being helpless and lost behind me once more.

That evening, just hours before check-in, Phil's girlfriend drove four of us: She, Phil, me, and Phil's sister as my fill-in date, in her dad's Thunderbird to see ***Psycho*** at a drive-in movie.

As she and Phil necked in the front seat, I did my best to carry on a conversation with his sister. She was good looking and deep down I always wished I had tried to kiss her. But I hardly had the self esteem to give it a try.

The next morning, again in the T-bird, the four of us traveled to the Marine base at Camp Pendleton. We would be there for 3 weeks, living in Quonset huts in the mountains during jungle warfare training.

The entrance to the base was visible in the distance as we parked at an observation-point above a cliff-lined lagoon. Phil and his girlfriend held each other and stared at the ocean. His sister and I shuffled about, trying not to look uncomfortable. I wondered if this might be the last girl I would touch in my life since there was a good chance I'd die in Vietnam. But I let the opportunity to kiss her, permission or not, slip away.

The drive from the lookout to the base seemed as if we had traveled at light speed, and within moments, Phil and I were walking through the main gate together.

****

Situated in the desolate mountains nicknamed *Las Pulgas* (the fleas in Spanish), several companies of Marines were prepared for jungle warfare, with fake villages and mock interrogations. There was even a demonstration on one frighteningly cold morning on how to kill and skin a rabbit following a karate-type blow by an instructor to the back of its neck.

The last night of our training, each man was disarmed and channeled single-file through a barbed wire portico where we'd simulate being captured. Just after sunset, teams of three were fed a cup-each of warm rice and led to an orchestrated "escape" route through the barbed wire.

Our goal that night was for each team to make their way through the mountains to a rendezvous point. Throughout the journey, we would use evasion techniques to avoid capture by Marine Reservists, also traveling in the hills, dressed as VC guerillas.

When my team finally made it to the comfort of a roaring fire I collapsed. Exhausted, I had fallen asleep so close to the flames that the blanket I had wrapped myself-in had caught fire.

The next few days were mostly unmemorable. One morning with little fanfare, my company was bussed to an airstrip where a commercial jet was waiting. Our destination was Okinawa.

The flight plodded-on and after nearly eight hours in the air I was elated as the U.S. Air Force base on the outskirts of Honolulu appeared below us.

On landing we scrambled to get off the plane and onto the tarmac, where we could stretch and catch a glimpse of Honolulu's skyline. But with barely enough time to smoke a cigarette, we re-boarded and were off to Okinawa where we'd get our first real taste of the orient and begin a slow, and for some, a painful acclimation to the heat.

On Okie; the island's nickname, we would among other things, store the bulk of our uniforms not needed in Nam in a second sea bag, which for reasons that seemed purposely cold and darkly efficient, we placed in a mammoth building among a literal sea of others. If we didn't make it back, we were told it would be sent home to our families.

From Kadena Air Base we ferried by cattle car; a sort of green city bus, from the airstrip to the Marine base. The sights and smells of Asia rattled my senses as we passed through the small roadside towns, walled on both sides of the dusty road with tightly packed rows of small shops. Nearly every storefront and kiosk along the route seemed to be held upright by patchworks of colorful metal signs, most of them advertising American soft drinks and cigarettes.

I was mesmerized by the strange varieties of food and bizarre products on display in each town. Now and then, many of us would gasp at the sight of a snake, as long as two men are tall and big around as a loaf of bread hanging from hooks outside a stall.

There weren't many occasions in the Corps when the adage of "hurry up and wait" didn't apply. But on Okie, the pace moved quickly, and before noon-chow our first day we were unloaded; assigned a bunk and marched to a metal building with rows and rows of neatly aligned, one-piece school-desks — the kind with a letter P shaped, one-piece writing surface and armrest attached to the chair.

We were ordered to find a seat and made quiet conversation about what might happen next.

Then through a side door at the front of the room, a giant Gunnery Sergeant appeared, quickly moving to a small stage.

The Gunny was terrifying, with a face as dark as coal and the strong features of his African heritage etched over his brow and along the geometry of both cheeks as if chiseled into a wodge of slate. Then with one giant leap, the Gunny landed with both feet atop a battered oak desk which growled beneath him.

The Gunny's message was simple and to the point:

"Marines," he bellowed. "Your fellow Marines need your blood to make it home. My job is to make sure that every swingin' dick that passes through this island gives his share," and he hesitated, slowly scanning the room with only his eyes as if to test the impact of his statement.

And then he roared: "Now who's gonna be the chicken-shit motherfucker who doesn't want to give blood today!"

Dead silence — Not one hand went up.

Satisfied, the Gunny jumped off the desk. He thanked us as he directed the first row to exit to his left and for each consecutive one to follow.

After each Marine had given his share of blood we were directed toward a hallway where a Navy Corpsman offered each man the choice of a shot of whisky in a small paper cup, or, an equally small portion of orange juice.

Since I was feeling very macho I said whisky and swallowed it in one fire-breathing gulp. A few steps further down the hallway another Corpsman handed each of us what would be our first malaria pill. Once "in-country" (Vietnam) it would be our Corpsman's responsibility to make sure we took one of the large orange tablets each Sunday.

No big deal — Right?

We went straight from the medical unit to noon-muster, aligning ourselves as always in precise columns in the blazing heat. In short time we'd be getting instructions for the remainder of the day.

Then without warning, my body fell forward in slow motion. As I collapsed, I pushed the Marine in front of me from the ranks, causing him to pivot-aside and provide me a clearing to land, unconscious, face-first on the lava-hot pavement.

I never made it to liberty that night. Evidently the combination of giving blood, drinking whisky and the malaria pill was too much. All I could do was lay in the rack the entire evening, as one-by- one the others returned to the squad bay; drunk as skunks; laughing and bragging about their first encounters with Asian girls.

As for me: my relief would be sleep, and the knowledge that in less than thirty-six hours we'd be on our way.

****

We arrived in DaNang, South Vietnam, in what else, but the heat of the afternoon.

It was only March, yet the humidity caused our starched uniforms to be soaked with sweat as we made our way from the airliner to an open-air terminal. It had a dirt floor and was covered with a wavy galvanized steel roof to block out the sun in summer and deter the months of incessant rain that would begin around Thanksgiving.

Inside, under cover by some standards, benches like church pews were scattered here and there, packed to capacity with young men in faded green jungle clothes. But there was nothing more in the way of accommodations. The atmosphere reminded me of how a railway station might look in some hell-hole like Bombay or Sri Lanka.

Most of us "new guys" gathered in small packs along the building's inside perimeter waiting for what would happen next.

We must have looked like hicks on their first visit to the big city; gawking as I did in awe of the hardened Marine grunts, barely a year older than I, and the infamous ROK (Republic of [South] Korea) Blue Dragons as they mulled about. And I imagined; no, I hoped, that if I made it back to this very spot, 13 months from this moment that new guys arriving would look at me with the same kind of wonder and admiration.

To the rear of the building, hundreds of shabby hooches extended across the vast compound for as far as I could see. Each small structure mirrored its counterpart, with a plywood deck suspended on legs thirty inches or so off the ground. A two feet tall plywood knee-wall was attached around their perimeters, topped with dust-caked screens extending to where the roof-gable attaches. Within each hooch, canvas cots were nudged close together along both long walls.

Sleep probably isn't the right term for how my first night in Nam went. The smells of the strange world outside the dusty screen were intoxicating — a combination of burning wood and stale beer; cigarettes and gunpowder; coffee and after shave; dirty feet and diesel fuel — a lot of diesel fuel!

I was glad Phil was still with me, and the next morning we went to chow together. We both were excited about the assignments we'd be getting. After a breakfast of hobo coffee, scrambled eggs and limp "hospital toast" we collected our in-country seabags and lined up in front of a small plywood shack not much bigger than a chicken coop.

As each Marine stepped forward and called out his name, an NCO, understandably grumpy and tired of the hundreds of questions by new guys every day, turned and fingered his way through a box of brown envelopes, slapping each one on the plywood counter with the same KER-PLUNK!

From there things happened so fast that before I knew it Phil was gone and I was alone.

"McGarrity, James M." I said and the Corporal plopped my envelope down in the same manner.

"You're going to Phu Bai," he said. "There's a plane leaving this afternoon."

"Next!"

I backed away from the shack and saw written across the front in black marker: 3d M.T. Battalion.

"Third what?

What does M.T. mean?

Mountain something?

Military something?"

I glanced at others' envelopes for a clue, but nothing made sense.

I returned to the shack and asked the Corporal what the initials meant.

I was confused when he told me.

"What?" I asked myself as I walked toward the flight line.

"M.T. stands for Motor Transport?"

But I'm a radio operator!"

"That's truck drivers and such — isn't it?"

3d Motors was based in Phu Bai, up north in the I Corps Military Tactical Zone. The Corporal said that a C-130 transport was preparing to depart for there and out on the runway I could see the plane's rear hatch yawned fully open and resting on the tarmac.

Inside, a jungle of orange straps dangled from the overhead forming a seat-of-sorts and I wiggled into one.

Soon more people entered and the harnesses quickly filled with passengers. It was obvious that many of them were new-guys like me — mostly Marines and a few Seabees, plus one or two U.S. Army soldiers.

Some of the passengers were dressed in dingy and disheveled dress-uniforms and through bloodshot eyes and poor shaves it was obvious that several were struggling with the effects of hangovers. I'd realize later that the worst-for-wear were returning from R&R (rest and recuperation) in Japan or Manila or Kuala Lumpur, where for up to a week, tiny brunettes in mini-skirts and high heels had made all their young fantasies come true.

As the plane roared over the city, the ramshackle rues and hovels of DaNang dotted the landscape toward the Hai Van Pass where Highway 1 zig-zags over the summit before dropping into a backdrop of emerald mountains and valleys.

As the tracts of jungle passed below us, I was distracted by the conspicuous prowling of the crew chief — an enlisted man who danced back-and-forth above us on a six-feet-tall metal bulkhead, slightly wider than a balance beam which ran the full length of the compartment.

Now and then the crew chief would come to a dead stop atop the wall. Then balancing himself with both hands clenched tightly on the nearest straps like a human marionette, he'd kneel and make wide-eyed expressions of concern through the portholes, followed by a loud, conspicuous conversation through his handset with some unseen crewman that I figured must have been one of the pilots.

I don't know — he may have been alerted to something.

But I've often thought, that if he was just B-S-ing us new guys to see our reactions —it worked!

****

By the time we approached the airstrip at Phu Bai it was pitch-black outside and the only light in the compartment came from several dull running-lamps in the overhead.

The plane powered-down as we drifted over the 3d Marine Division's eastern perimeter, where around the clock, Marines and Navy Seabees manned an endless series of sandbagged trenches and precisely-spaced wooden towers, forty feet tall.

Dropping deeper through the darkness, the flying boxcar shuddered as its flaps plowed the night air. Here and there, illumination flares could be seen floating indiscriminately around the perimeter, revealing ghostly, phosphorescent images of an occasional Marine or sailor moving along beaten paths connecting the bunkers.

And then with one mighty plunge and a blast of counter propulsion we hit the runway and rolled to a stop.

As the rear hatch hissed open I could see beyond the pale red glow of the interior a small shack at the edge of the field. A single light bulb dangled from the ceiling illuminating the silhouette of a human figure.

As I followed fellow travelers down the ramp, the crew chief, having noticed my brown, new-guy envelope, said as I passed him that the guy in the shack would call my outfit to pick me up.

I thanked him and as my eyes went to night-vision in the darkness, I could see the moonlit outline of a pyramid-shaped mountain in the distance.

Suddenly from atop the mountain bursts of red tracers cut downward through the night, passing green ones rocketing upward. Other volleys ricocheted off boulders and catapulted into the black abyss of heaven.

Alone in the darkness of the airstrip I watched the battle unfold.

Then it occurred to me:

“Damn! That’s a firefight!”

“Man,” I thought, “This is one hell of a long way from home!”

I continued my way toward the shack where I showed my orders to a tired guard. He cranked the handle of a battery operated field phone and told a garbled and equally sleepy-sounding voice on the other end that a “new guy” was reporting in.

In no time at all, a growling rectangular shadow guided by two strips of light, came to a stop just inches from me.

I climbed into the open rear seat of the Jeep and introduced myself to its two ghostly occupants. They answered briefly and we sped off through the night.

About a mile from the airstrip the Jeep approached a tiny guard shack where a figure with a rifle signaled for us to stop. Recognizing the driver, the guard removed a flimsy barricade and waved us in.

Within seconds we were parked outside a hooch very similar to the one I spent my first night in at DaNang.

The three of us entered and in a halo of candlelight I could see silhouettes here and there on canvas cots. One of the guys from the Jeep pointed me toward an empty one. I was exhausted and glad to finally get some rest.

Laying there in the darkness there was something familiar; almost comforting in the smells seeping through the screen beside me, like when my cousin and I would sleep-out as kids; Smells like old plywood and musty canvas and the last wisp of smoke from a dying fire.

And once again, I fell into a deep sleep.

The following morning I awoke to the sounds of a dozen radios resonating throughout the compound. There were eight cots inside the hooch but only three appeared as if they were slept in. One of the guys introduced himself and volunteered to show me where the chow tent was. He told me that after we ate he'd take me to meet Sergeant B and he handed me a dull stainless steel tray with a larger than normal fork and knife and spoon attached to it with a heavy piece of electrical wire.

There's no telling how long I had rehearsed the speech, but as soon as I got a chance I told Sergeant B how concerned I was about using Code.

Radio telegraph school had drilled some real hard-Corps responsibility into us, about how hundreds of Marines would depend on us to get them medical help or call for reinforcements or air support to save our butts.

But frankly, the prospect of that sort of responsibility scared me to death. I didn't know it then, but I believe my terror regarding responsibility was tied to my self esteem, which was destroyed on a picture-perfect summer day in 1962, when I was 15.

****

I was staying with my cousin in the country, as I often did. My mother had remarried three years earlier and I was told that her new husband said the drive to his business in the city was too far. Evidently it was especially far from the little house in the country where my mother and I had lived with my grandmother.

At first I gave in; he seemed like a good enough guy and had more money than anyone from the dirt back road. Besides, deep in my heart-of-hearts I believed that the move to a rented apartment in the city was only temporary, and soon we'd return to the country, living in a fine new home better than any that my friends on the back road had. I imagined, how from my new and privileged life, I could ride my bike to see my cousin and my friends any time I wanted.

Even throughout our first months in the city, I never gave up on my belief that it was only a matter of time until we returned to the country.

But we didn't move back— we moved even further — clear to the other side of the city.

A year later, at thirteen, I still hated life in the city, with its tough looking kids and fights after school and funny ideas — like a boy in junior high who rode a bike was weird.

I loved riding bikes! They could take you anywhere you wanted to go.

What's weird about that? I guess my feelings were obvious. So much so that I'm positive my mother understood that I felt like an outsider so she seldom refused my pleas on weekends to haul me and my bike to my cousin's house on the dirt back road for weekend visits.

By the time I reached ninth grade, I still longed for the simple joys of the country, where how you dressed and acted didn't matter, and where late into the night, my cousin and me and our friends would build bonfires and roast corn and sleep-out in old junk cars, laughing like fools and smoking rolled-cigarettes and cussing till the fire went out. And with the embers glowing red in the darkness, the bunch of us would fall asleep under nappy blankets with no more on our minds than what tomorrow would bring.

It was on such a morning that my cousin and I decided that if we helped a friend deliver his newspapers, we'd have more time to enjoy the day, so the three of us rode our bicycles to the main highway. We had already decided to split the route — my cousin and our friend going to the right — and me to the left.

Just minutes up the road I reached the last house and threw the paper onto the porch. I coasted down the cinder drive toward the main highway. I could see the last houses on the opposite side that would finish the route, and thought how it wouldn't be long before I met up with the others.

I looked right — I'm positive I looked to my left. I'm sure I would have; We spent a lot of time riding the busy highway tributaries connecting the neighborhoods of the back road had learned early-on the rules and dangers of the road.

Everything seemed fine, and I pedaled toward the center line.

Then suddenly I wasn't riding my bicycle anymore.

Everything was dark.

I could feel blades of grass tickling the backs of my arms from my elbows to my wrists.

Why was I on my back?

There were voices all around me — adult voices, and I thought how strange it was that dinner-time was hours away, yet it was dark outside and I couldn't move and there was a warm, thick fluid of some sort streaming over both cheeks. It was then that I had a frightening sense that something was wrong as a cool breeze wafted over my face and cold streams ran down and dripped-off the back of my neck as synchronous as rain washes down a gutter.

I was transported at breathtaking speed to Children's Hospital in a red Cadillac ambulance. Its siren howled like a banshee and sunlight ricocheted throughout the interior as the powerful car rocketed-by trees and rooftops.

A man in the Cadillac squeezed-in beside the gurney where I laid and pressed his hand against my carotid artery the entire way to town.

The last thing I remember was the smell of antiseptic and stern voices all around me as my pants were stripped off.

"Oh no," I thought. "I hope my Mom doesn't see I had a pack of cigarettes in my pocket."

Then everything was black again for a long time. I envisioned that I was floating in space and in the distance were two tiny lights; at first looking like stars. But then the stars came toward me, faster and faster, until in a flash they were inches away.

For a brief moment I saw that they were the headlights of a car. Then a blinding CRASH!

The explosion was followed over and over by darkness — deep space — and the headlights returning.

Three days later I regained consciousness.

My mother was sitting at my bedside with one arm on my leg and her head resting atop it.

I reached out and my hand fell on her thick, perfect black hair.

“What happened?” I mumbled.

She moved her face close to mine and spent several moments taking in the reality of it all.

“You were in a terrible accident,” she whispered.

“You were hit by a car and went through the windshield,” and she paused, as if saying the next few words would be the hardest thing she would ever do in her life.

In the end, they were:

“And your face — was terribly cut,” she whispered.

Then she held my hand against her lips and she cried.

Later that day, when no one was around, I slowly traced the roadmap of stitches on my face with one finger. I was told that there were a lot of them, but I never could have imagined there were so many. Along with the stitches, my nose was packed with gauze as all the cartilage that formed the bridge had been destroyed and my front teeth had been pushed up against the roof of my mouth. But an incredible reconstructive surgeon, Dr. Sol Braver of the Ewing Clinic in Akron repositioned them as I lay near death on the emergency room table. The only other visible injuries were large circular road-rash burns on my right shoulder and leg from where I rolled off the hood and slid across the road.

I was a mess.

A perfect summer morning delivering newspapers had changed my life in seconds

I believe it’s the reason why for so many years I hated life and everyone in it: Everyone who got better grades; everyone who was a jock or popular; everyone who was handsome or thought they were, or any one of a thousand other reasons.

I didn’t die that day — but my self esteem did.

I had become a victim.

I was worthless.

****

Responsibility!

They'd all be depending on me to save them?

Are you crazy?

Just give me a gun and let me kill some VC!

That's all I want to do!

But the Marines don't work that way. They decide what you're best suited for and by God, that's what you'll do!

For some crazy reason the Corps had decided that I'd be a good communicator.

Obviously, having taken three years of French and the very-real possibility that I'd be going to a country where French was a second language, you'd think I had skills that could make me an interpreter or something.

But the Corps had decided that I should learn Morse code.

In the end I did alright with code. But the training was mentally burdening.

To graduate we were required to receive 12 words a minute — that's one letter; called a character; every second.

So for 16 weeks, hour after hour, day after day, five days a week, we listened to code through headsets in outdated, two story wood buildings in the middle of summer with the only moving air from old reciprocating fans.

To top it off, every week there was a test, with each student required to achieve a higher proficiency in word-count. If you failed, you packed your gear, left everyone you had made friends with, and moved-in with the class behind you to pick-up and re-qualify where you failed.

If you were unable to pass the next word-count test — then you went backward again!

There were no transfers or quitting. The only way out was the brig or the mental ward.

And so with each passing week the pressure increased.

"You'll have to save lives!" the instructors told us.

"Everyone will depend on you!"

"What?" I thought. "Me save lives!"

“But we were trained to take lives!”

“Damn! I don’t know if I can do this code stuff!”

But there was no way out.

I would have to do it.

I would have to save them.

It would all be up to me.

But using Morse code?

How?

Sure, I was fine at transmitting.

I seemed to have a knack for it and my finger danced on the key:

Dit-dit-dit — Daw-daw-daw — Dit- dit-dit: for SOS.

But I was struggling with the rising word-count and so were many of my classmates.

Some of them became so obsessed with copying messages at the higher speeds that they bought tape recorders; taping sessions during the day and playing them back through earphones while they were asleep.

At night in the squad-bay I could hear my classmates mumbling the sing-song cadence of code in their sleep:

*"**Dit-dit-dit — Dit-dit-dit.**"*

I even heard that some who could afford it were getting hypnotized.

But save lives?

Under fire?

How could I ever do that?

So the first thing after chow that first morning in Nam I cornered Sergeant B and recited the speech I had rehearsed since leaving Okinawa.

We were standing in front of the old French bunker we used for a communication shack when I confessed my fears to him.

Then Sergeant B said:

"You're never gonna use that code crap here," he said.

And he walked away.

"Thank you God," I thought to myself.

II

OLD SARGE

March turned to June yet I remained, with no animosity a "new guy." That meant that I would continue to be assigned as communicator on the mine truck.

Thankfully, by this period in the war, the only incidents our battalion encountered were from the occasional generic road mines. These less devastatingly charged explosives seemed designed to blow a wheel or fender off and mostly disrupt us.

I'd say we were fortunate that no one in our communications' platoon had been seriously wounded, though one of our guys did get a Purple Heart when some road gravel from a land mine peppered the underside of his arm.

This particular June morning I had pulled the 12 to 4 AM watch. Having been an especially boring four hours, and with no need to debrief my replacement, I left the bunker and walked alone through the morning darkness.

Passing silently among the rows of hooches, the only signs of life, other than the occasional moan or snort of someone asleep were the subtle glow of landing lights and roars of C-130's coming-and-going at the Phu Bai airstrip. Their distinctive around-the-clock commotions had become strangely comforting, and no sooner had I stretched out on my cot than I drowned in sleep.

At sunrise I awoke to the same sights as every other day; Vietnam's pitiful main highway — Highway 1, bustling with a never-ending parade of peasants and scooters and stray dogs; ARVN soldiers dodging overloaded micro-buses; barefoot mama-sans and water buffaloes on their way to God knows where, somehow managing to keep from trampling each other in the process.

I imagined how in a very short time I'd be joining them, heading north to Camp Evans or Dong Ha or Quang Tri; maybe even as far as Khe Sanh; delivering the precious cargoes of ammunition and food and clothing and everything imaginable that our fellow Marines in the remote camps and firebases of I Corps (First Corps but pronounced in military jargon like the letter i) relied-on for their daily survival.

I could also see that a dozen or so trucks had already assembled in the staging area, a hundred yards or so beyond our wire. As I dressed, my plan after morning chow was to hitch a ride to staging with whoever would be driving the convoy commander. The two of them, plus our battalion Corpsman, would be following in a Jeep a short distance behind the truck's driver and me in the lead vehicle.

I'd be traveling light — no rifle today — just my Colt sidearm and some extra magazines of .45 caliber ammo.

I grabbed two packs of Marlboros and rifled through a cardboard C-rations' container for a single meal in case the field mess at Camp Evans was closed when we arrived. Finding a Beefsteak and Potatoes, I dropped the small cardboard box and its contents of canned fruit and John Wayne crackers (a dry, round, saltine of sorts) into my laundry- sack-sized waterproof bag.

The Beefsteak was packed in a soup-sized can and was easy to heat. Occasionally I'd nuzzle the container somewhere in the engine compartment, so when we arrived it would be hot. Other times I might use a marble-sized ball of C-4 explosive (when lit it doesn't explode but burns like mad) or a commercial Sterno-like heat tablet. When neither of those was available, I'd make an improvised stove in a smaller can by pouring a little diesel fuel over some dirty pebbles sprinkled in the bottom. The stones seemed to stifle the dark smoke and soot buildup.

My driver in the mine truck this particular morning was a BNG; a brand new guy, from somewhere I never heard of. It was apparent from the moment we met that the possibility of being blown-to-hell by a road mine had him worried.

I told him that duty on the truck sounded worse than it actually was and that the VC (Viet Cong) had quickly learned that the lead truck of a convoy, with nothing more valuable onboard than several hundred pounds of sandbags and two lowly Privates, was a waste of good explosives. As a result of this, I continued, seemed to emerge a revised tactic of using more command-operated detonators instead of pressure-detonated ones, which relied on us to roll over them.

This strategy I added, allowed the VC to pick their targets at will. It made our convoys sitting ducks for a sapper to lay in hiding and position their explosives in a mound of dirt or ditch or pothole. Then all it took was to wait for the perfect opportunity to take-out something vital.

My observations didn't seem to ease him much, for as he pulled onto the highway, he ground the gears as if it was his first time behind the wheel, coaxing wide grins from two Vietnamese

Provincial Force (PF) sentries manning a crude roadside bunker.

This was our first checkpoint. It was the first of many we would pass this day.

Time to go to work!

"Beach Boy Actual" I said into the handset: "This is Beach Boy Advance — Over."

"Actual" was the convoy commander's call sign.

"Advance" was my call sign in the mine truck.

"Be advised we are departing Checkpoint Seven," I said, and my counterpart replied with a simple yet distinctive and purposeful: "Rrr...oger, Advance;" emphasizing the rolling cadence of his r's as most of us did.

Our first key destination would be the ancient imperial capital of Hue, about 10 miles north of Phu Bai and setting of the brutal house-to-house fighting that would take place soon during the 1968 Tet Offensive (Lunar New Year) in January.
Hue was the treasure of Vietnamese culture for centuries, and even after Saigon became the capitol, Hue remained a bustling, jungle-brimmed metropolis, with banks, museums, a deluxe French-built hotel, a university and a resplendent catholic cathedral.

Approaching Hue from Phu Bai, Highway1; barely two lanes wide and consisting primarily of asphalt-filled potholes and tamped-gravel, sits atop a great earthen dike. Broad plains of rice paddies extend from each side of the embankment as far as the eye can see to the East, and to the threshold of an emerald-green jungle to our left.

Foot travelers and vehicles nearing the city are funneled through a concrete and fresco archway, then toward a dusty fountain in the center of a roundabout, where ox-paths and foot trails converge on the circle like spokes on a wheel.

As we rounded the fountain, each vehicle churned a cloud of dust, engulfing the pool's bullet-riddled and neglected whitewashed wall.
From the circle it's a straight drive north toward the heart of the city, where Thuy Dan Street, a Parisian-like boulevard of flowering trees and intoxicating aromas parallels the ancient Perfume River.

At the west end of the boulevard we climb a rise and turn north onto Checkpoint 2-6 (26): one of two leviathan iron bridges spanning the river, thanks to years of French engineering and hard labor under the boot of colonialism.

"Beach Boy Actual," I said, as the truck bucked onto the wooden deck.

"Be advised we are crossing Checkpoint 2-6," and the radioman driving the C.O. confirmed my message.

As the driver picked his way across the planks, I checked the chamber of my .45 and slid it into its holster. In minutes we'd be entering the Viet Cong's domain; north of Hue, where civilians hurried-by in dingy black pajamas; their faces cast downward to avoid eye contact, and where children line the roadsides in every village begging us to toss them a can of C-rations or anything for that matter to convert into money for their own use or to pay off VC "tax collectors."

"Hey you, Marine — Marine Number 1," they'd call, and give us the thumbs up.

"You give me C's?" (c-rations) they'd say.

When we didn't throw them something they'd give us the middle finger and holler:

"Fuck you Marine! — Marine number 10!"

Which meant of course — "You no good!"

One thing I quickly learned about the Vietnamese — they aren't bashful, as toughness is part of their DNA. If you want proof, consider that they've been killing and dying since the days of the Tonkin Dynasty, when they repelled

Kublai Khan not once — but twice!

Then in the 1940's, while Japan was occupying Burma and Malaysia and the Philippines by force, Japan's Emperor opted against military confrontation with Vietnam en-lieu of negotiations; Probably a smart move on the Japanese's part.

Then in the 1950's, the Viet Minh (League for the Independence of Vietnam) defeated the French Army at the Battle of Dien Bien Phu despite the ferocity of a battalion of French Legionnaires, who many, including myself, regard as some of the toughest soldiers on earth.

Dien Bien Phu became the hallmark for the mistakes of entrenched defenses:

"Never Take The Low Ground!"

Unfortunately, America repeated the same mistake at Khe Sanh, even though those of us who were there never lost a battle and defended the American outpost under tremendous artillery barrages, until the generals and U.S. politicians shut it down.

****

With Checkpoint 2-6 behind us, our convoy was about five miles north of Hue where the terrain becomes a sandy flatland spattered with small communities of thatched huts; scrub-grass; streams and backwater canals.

It was about here that I began receiving garbled, nearly indecipherable transmissions on the PRC-10 radio I was issued that morning.

PRC stands for Portable Radio Communications and as far as I was concerned, the PRC-10 and its counterparts, the PRC-8 and PRC-9 were about as worthless a piece of communication gear as was ever invented.

Whenever I got stuck with one of these Korean War era poor excuses for a radio, I'd scrounge-up a squawk box: a 4" square externally attachable speaker that I would place on the seat beside me. At least with this I felt I could better hear and decipher who was trying to contact me.

The squawk box has about a three feet long rubber cord which allows it to be plugged-in and set within hearing distance. This day, as I often did, I placed it on the seat between me and the driver where it danced in unison to the potholes.

A few miles north of Hue, it's necessary to cross a mile-long section of roadway elevated above an immense rice paddy.

I had my attention focused on a group of trees, 100 meters or so in the distance to my left. It was an oasislooking, almost idyllic setting with tall trees sheltering a small village. I was focusing my attention toward the village when a Huey helicopter appeared over the wood-line to my right. It was flying low at a high rate of speed straight toward the village.

It was then that I heard a transmission crackle from the squawk box. It sounded something like: "(indiscernible)…….a firefight," or maybe, that's how I want to remember the voice having said.

Or was it that I wanted to screw with the new kid?

Or maybe I wanted to break the boredom of the miles passing-by?

Who knows?

But nothing throughout the nagging years of replaying that day, changes the fact that the driver had been frightened that morning — and I knew it.

Then the driver heard me say:

"I think I heard something like a firefight ahead," and he blurted-out something. Obviously alarmed, the driver tried to grab the speaker with his right hand while steering with his left.

I guess he just wanted to hear it for himself.

Then wouldn't you know — the speaker fell on the floor.

Again the driver reached for it — even further — but now his head was below his field of vision.

"I'll get it! — I'll get it!" I shouted.

But he kept trying to grab it!

That's when I felt the truck tipping to the right; crunching and sliding in the gravel beside the road until gravity and the point-of-no-return pulled the truck into a dive.

And then I was weightless.

My last sight of the driver was his ass-end as he leaped out the door just as the truck and I disappeared over the edge.

When I regained my senses I was inside the overturned cab — neck-deep in foul water. Unable to move, I was pinned in a death grip of sandbags, which seconds earlier had lined the floor and became dislodged as the truck tumbled upside down.

Stunned and disoriented, my first fears weren't of drowning, but of the truck catching fire or that a snake; maybe a cobra, as they often nest along banks, might be whipping-about searching for its own escape.

Then I heard voices and the sloshing sounds of boots in the water as Marines began pulling the soaked bags off me.

In no time I was free and being helped up the bank to the road. I was covered with dark, dung-sopped water, but otherwise, I didn't seem to have any injuries.

There was a somber mood when we reached the road. I could see several Marines gathered in a circle, looking down at something on the pavement.

It was a person for sure — a Marine.

I expected it to be the driver, but as I moved closer I was shocked by the sight of our beloved battalion Master Sergeant, flat on his back, broken and twisted and struggling for his last breath. His farewell his last day on earth, after decades of service to the Corps, was signaled with a jagged bone, red and ivory and dotted with flies. The bone protruded from a ragged rip in his forearm, waving a tiny gesture with each breath.

And that's when it hit me.

He had been riding in the open bed of our truck.

I didn't know he was there!

He seldom left the compound!

"Oh my God!"

When the truck flipped, he must have been thrown off — or jumped!

"Is this my fault?" I asked myself.

The uncertainty; the guilt; hit me like lightning.

There was no way around it.

If I hadn't said that thing about the firefight, the driver wouldn't have panicked and the Sarge would still be alive.

****

I don't remember much about the rest of that day or many days afterward to tell the truth.

The word around camp in the days following the accident was that he had been flown to Guam and was still alive — but in very bad shape
Eight to ten days later it was official — he had died.

A Navy chaplain came to our compound and held a brief ceremony for him. I stood at the back of the tent as the padre began the memorial. He said something like:

“Blah, blah, blah ....Master Sergeant P has gone to meet the Great Commandant in the sky.”

“No! He couldn’t be saying that!” I said to myself.

“He couldn’t be saying that God is a Marine!”

****

Dusk was falling on the mountain that captivated me that first night on the airstrip, and I glanced its way as the tent-flap folded behind me and I walked off — alone — feeling as bad as I ever had in my life.

I yearned for the guys in my platoon to say something — Anything!
Please, give me some sign that the Sarge’s death wasn’t my fault!

But they didn’t.

We never said anything to each other about deaths on the road:

We’d get high on weed — sometimes we got drunk — other times we went to sleep.

But we never talked about it.

Several days later, a legal officer from 3d Division interviewed me about the Sarge's death.

I was scared to the point of vomiting that I would be blamed and barely slept for days beforehand.

In the end, it must have been determined that it was the driver's fault, because I never saw him around the compound afterward.

I hoped with all my heart that he wouldn't get court-martialed.

I guess I could have taken more blame for what happened.

But I didn't.

It was cruel but true in Nam: the only atonement available: But for some crazy reason it worked — at least we thought it did. It was summed-up in five simple words:

"Ain't nothin' but a thing."

III

Thirty-Nine Five

The death of our battalion Master Sergeant triggered an unshakable obsession within me for safety. Not my safety, but a deep-seeded fixation on the life-and-death responsibilities I was charged with. For I had made a covenant the evening of the Sarge's memorial, that never again would someone die because of something I did, or didn't do.

Like many things sworn-to on impulse or emotion, the power driving a vow can be ruthless. For every day, at least two or three of the guys in my platoon — myself included, were on the road providing support. One of us would drive the convoy commander with the battalion Corpsman crammed-into the small back seat. Then of course, another radioman would ride in the cab of the point vehicle — the mine truck.

On larger convoys, as an array of operational vehicles tagged-along loaded with everything from artillery-rounds to grunts (Marine riflemen), a third radioman would bring up the rear in our old but reliable MRC-83 Jeep. It had a monstrous UHF radio that filled what would have normally been a back seat and a towering fiberglass antenna which we looped in an arc over the canvas canopy and secured with a cord to the front bumper.

The MRC-83's powerful-looking antenna and coffin-sized radio was in reality a paper-tiger. On one hand, it could pick up propaganda from Hanoi Hannah or garbled chatter from as far away as Hawaii. But otherwise, it was useless for transmitting from even the front to the rear of a convoy.

The Jeep's one great asset however was its ability to dig its way, submerged, through water. And I drove one quite a few times from landing craft, with nothing more than my head cutting through the surf and a smoking exhaust-pipe-extension chattering behind me like a hot periscope.

****

Around July, 1967, a series of convoys took us deep into the Ashau Valley to support the Fourth Marine Regiment — possibly the 1st Battalion. They were memorable to me for their call-sign: *Mary Jane*; slang, at least to us enlisted guys, for marijuana.

One Company of One/Four: (the phonetic abbreviation for First Battalion/Fourth Marines [1/4]), was set-up on two barren hills, smack-dab in the deepest jungle. The outpost included a small U.S. Army artillery crew manning a 175 mm cannon. To accommodate the massive artillery-piece, the canopy which had camouflaged the two mounds from time immemorial had been stripped of all life with defoliants. These were the same chemicals acknowledged years later as being responsible for the laundry list of illnesses plaguing Vietnam vets.

Penetrating the jungle roads and ambush-rich passes of the Ashau Valley to reach the evolving outposts took our mission to a new level. I realize now, that in many ways we had become conditioned to the attacks against us on Highway 1, regardless of injuries becoming more numerous and lethal. Despite the rising destructive powers of VC explosives, at least on the somewhat exposed surroundings of the main road we had a better view of the terrain and field of fire.

But now the enemy was all around us — up close and personal.

These were the real bad guys: the NVA — North Vietnamese Army regulars who operated the miles of underground tunnels and weapons' caches and where doctors performed surgery in hand-carved caverns lit by kerosene lanterns.

At one camp deep in the jungle, Marine reconnaissance reported that at least on one occasion while "snoopin' and poopin'" near the Ho Chi Minh Trail, not far from us, they could hear the low-pitched drone of Russian-made trucks.

Understandably, this period in the war marked the time when American losses were reaching enormous proportions. Three quarters of the way through 1967 alone, American combat deaths surpassed 10,000, mostly nineteen and twenty-year-olds.

For us, escalation of harm meant road mines of increasing power and we went from explosives meant to slow us down, to powerful munitions capable of sending our heavy trucks cartwheeling end-over-end.

It was a frightening sight as vehicles just yards ahead of me landed upside down with their drivers trapped or unconscious inside as fuel ran in streams onto the roadway and artillery shells broken loose from their bundles, reeled through the spilled gasoline like deadly versions of spin-the-bottle.

Once, on a section of dirt road leading into the Ashau Valley, while plowing ankle-deep through an unnatural red powder — maybe Agent Orange — vehicles returning from the jungle passes exploded within yards of me on the oncoming side.

Increasing; frightening; and life-altering events had become an everyday occurrence.

I never gave much thought to the number of blast concussions I was experiencing and their physical toll. Corpsmen then I've been told were trained to triage under obvious factors — like bleeding — or burns. But evidently, their rule-of-thumb for a concussion during triage recommended that if a man's helmet was blown off, chances were he had a concussion.

Problem was — most of the time on the road I didn't wear a helmet.

I was about to see firsthand what the effects of ignoring our protective gear would mean, as once supplies were running successfully and regularly into the Ashau, others of us were diverted north.

On one of these new runs we were was just south of Camp Evans in Thua Thien (twa-tien) Province; north of Hue, when one of our vehicles was struck by an explosive device of some kind.

It was the biggest yet!

We were near this little village where a lot of VC activity took place, and over the past weeks, there had been a rash of harassing incidents here against us. Especially at a small bridge designated Checkpoint 14, or in communication jargon,so as not to be misunderstood: Checkpoint One-Four.

There was a legend regarding the Thua Thien area that it was haunted. It was even said that the Ninth Marines, when dug-in at night, would hear the sounds of specters whispering in chilling unison as they darted through the branches above them.

Maybe they were right! Hell, maybe the whole stinkin' province was evil! After all, Vietnam was a place of ancient and arcane mysteries.

Consider the accounts of writer Bao Ninh in his novel of everyday life in war from the communist soldier's experience, titled: *The Sorrow of War*. In his book, Ninh tells in frightening details of fellow fighters hearing similar sounds, especially in a place they called: The Jungle of Screaming Souls. Ninh also documented physical encounters claimed by comrades with corpses of countrymen as well as Americans, allegedly without heads, walking single file through the jungle with lanterns held above them.

And so in my mind, it wouldn't seem unusual, or for that matter, justifiable, that after numerous incidents against us, especially at the bridge, that I would become convinced that the entire village right down to the last pig and chicken was evil. And that meant, that death for any or all of them was irrelevant.

How else, time after time, could we keep getting the crap blown out of us, with people killed and wounded? Why was the village still standing? Hell, the Ninth Marines were only a few clicks away —Those bad-asses would burn it to the ground just for the practice.

Yet there it was: day after day; dirty, colorless; surrounded by pools of buffalo shit and splintered and stained bamboo poultry pens.

I was facing my biggest challenge yet, with two Marines seriously wounded from the blast and in need of medevac. Usually this was done by helicopter, or if deep in the field, by one of our battalion Otters; a super-light, rubber-tracked vehicle conceived in the 1950's for use in the polar-regions but found ideal for the wet terrain of Vietnam.

These young Marines needed evacuated — and needed it now!

Fortunately, one of the last original guys who showed me the ropes my first months in-country was driving the convoy commander this day, and amidst the chaos of a lot of people calling for help, he called to me that he'd get the choppers on the way.

Then he called to me to dial my radio to the MEDEVAC frequency: Thirty Nine-Five, and direct the medical evacuation choppers to the LZ.

"OK, I can do this." And I ran over the details in my mind of what needed to happen:

OK.

"One: Establish an LZ, a Landing Zone;"

"Two: Contact the pilot;"

"Three: Throw the smoke;"

"Four: Ask the pilot to confirm the color of the smoke;"

"DON'T FORGET THAT JIM! I said to myself.

SAY: "DO YOU SEE MY SMOKE!"

"ALWAYS ASK THE PILOT TO CONFIRM MY SMOKE!" —
"Remember what the guys told you about how Viet Cong radiomen will listen-in and throw the same color smoke if you announce it first!"

"That can bring the choppers into an ambush!

Damn!"

"OK, OK, what's the frequency?" I asked myself.

"Hey Jerry, what's the frequency?" I called to him.

He didn't hear me.

"Hey Jerry," I repeated. "What's the frequency?"

"39 — Five," he answered.

"OK," I thought: "39 — Five."

Frantically I ran the left knob to 39 and the right knob to zero-five.

How much clearer could it be — a 39 and a point zero-five.

The radio crackled and I strained to hear some indication from the pilot that he was near.

Nothing!

Then I heard Jerry's voice calling to me:

"There's the chopper Jim!" he hollered, pointing northward.

I seemed to be doing everything right!

I had a smoke canister ready to throw — there was background noise on the frequency — and I continued trying to contact the pilot:

"Delta Med — this is Beach Boy — Do you copy? — Over," I said.

Damn! He's getting closer!

"Come on — answer"!

"Delta Med, this is Beach Boy," I repeated.

"Do you copy? — Over," I said again.

"C'mon dammit — answer! I can't throw the smoke till you answer!"

I imagined a VC eavesdropper just beyond the tree line; peeking from a hole in the ground; listening; waiting; hoping that the hesitant young Marine would announce the color of the smoke so he could throw the same color himself. That could lead the choppers into an ambush. It would be my fault!

"Delta Med — Come in!" I pleaded.

"Why is he hovering, Jim?" Jerry hollered.

"I can't reach him!" I said.

Suddenly I heard the mechanical WHUMP-WHUMP-WHUMP of the medevac as it appeared on the ridgeline. I could see the pilot's silhouette in the cockpit. I slipped-out of my radio-pack and let it swing from one shoulder to the ground. I repeated the frequency I was dialed-in on back to Jerry:

"Thirty Nine point Zero-Five! — Right Jerry?" I hollered.

"You're on the wrong frequency," he answered. "It's 39 point Five-Zero; not 39 point Zero-Five!"

What! That's how it's read? And I ran the dials to the correct frequency.

By then Jerry had the microphone of the Jeep's more powerful RC-524 radio held close to his mouth with one hand and was motioning for me to throw the smoke with the other.

I pulled the ring from the smoke grenade and tossed it. As the smoke rose I heard the pilot confirm the color to Jerry and he dropped downward into the haze, blowing it in scattered billows in every direction.

I was humiliated.

I had done it again!

I had betrayed the vow — the vow that no one would die because of my errors.

"What if they died?

What if Jerry hadn't been here and I wouldn't have been able to reach the pilot because of a stupid, lousy mistake like missing something as simple as how to interpret a frequency."

On that day, at that moment, the promise I made to myself weeks earlier when our Master Sergeant died, echoed in my mind, and I repeated them with a resolve as duty bound as a curse-of-death as its consequence.

The words would have gone something like this:

"I swear that from this day on, I will be the best radioman there is. No one will ever have to fear not being saved when I'm with them. I will never be caught without the correct information again. No matter what the circumstances, I will not fail. I will never again face the possibility of letting my fellow Marines down. No matter what is needed --- I will do."

Something else happened that day. I thought I knew what anger and hatred were. But I learned of hatred that day that makes all others seem pale.

And so my second pledge went something like this:

"From this day on, I will kill the first person from that stinking village that I see near this bridge, so that I will never again face the possibility of letting my brothers down."

I'd soon have the opportunity to make that oath a reality, as by the time September rolled around, all but two of the original guys that were my mentors since March had rotated home, including our third platoon Sergeant.

By this point in my tour, mostly new guys made-up the bulk of our platoon. Now I was the one teaching *them* the ropes. I had become what I promised myself a month earlier — the best they had. Now officers were *asking* for me to be their radioman.

With the departure of Sergeant Montgomery, a new platoon sergeant arrived. Sergeant Morello was from 3d Recon and from day-one he turned us into a professional, powerful and respected unit; completely in charge of communicating in the field as officers often regarded us as pack mules — relegated to trudging alongside them; hauling our weapons; canteens; utility belt and extra batteries, while they stuck close-by, yakking nonprocedural B.S. into the handset.

But Sgt. Morello made it known in explicit terms that *his* men operated the radios, and on one occasion, he went as far as to belly-up to the battalion commander — a Major, that I, a lowly Lance Corporal had instructed to relinquish the handset to his radioman. It was a dicey decision for sure, but I felt boldly justified, albeit impulsive, when I heard him compromise one of our checkpoint's location on the air.

A bad decision? I wonder if in some dark domain of pre-consciousness, my decision was brought-on by the recent vow; A vow placing me as a savior in the face of suffering; A vow with rationality to me, but conceived in a mind where safety and the avoidance of guilt pairs with dire finality on the smallest detail, such as the slip of a tongue. Perhaps it was then, that it's true; that an altered-state had already taken place within me; A change in my thinking where the least miscalculation or lapse in judgment allowed no variables in consequence, except death or degradation.

The day at hand, I was in the communication bunker when the convoy returned. I had just received word that the commander's vehicle had entered the compound when heavy footsteps rattled the plank floor. It was the battalion commander.

As the Major entered the room I jumped to attention. I could see from the look on his face that I was about to get the ass-chewing of the century.

But Sergeant Morello was on the Major's heels and before he could get a word out, Sgt. M stepped between us.

"Sir," the Sarge said in a distinct, but not over-acted New Jersey accent.

"With all due respect sir, I believe Colonel (un-recollected) at Division Intelligence would be very concerned if he knew that one of our checkpoints was compromised?"

Major Stahl grimaced and stomped out of the bunker.

I learned later that the Major was aware that Sgt. Morello was privy to the facts of an embarrassing friendly-fire incident he was admonished-for while assigned as an artillery officer when he first arrived in-country.

The cards it appeared were in Sergeant M's favor, as they always seemed to be. He had been in Vietnam since 1965 when the 26th Marines landed at DaNang. During the next two years he rose through the ranks of the elite Marine Recon, with associates in Division Intelligence. He was one of those guys who "walked-the-walk" and once told me in private about a terrifying and celebrated operation into the mountains above Phu Loc: a Marine outpost constantly hit by enemy mortars. The mountains were a religious snactuary, which meant no incursion — at least officially.

After Sgt. M's team and a cadre of mercenaries made a midnight visit to the mountain, the mortars stopped.

In fact, everything stopped.

It was Sgt. Morello who taught me the power of communications and the awesome responsibility we were charged with when under attack.

RESPONSIBILITY!

There's that word again.

It had always been a feared circumstance for me.

Yet under Sgt. M it defined me!

For the first time in my adult life I was feeling good about myself — I was doing everything right — I was no longer the pathetic childhood victim of a terrible accident with a roadmap of scars on his face and a nose like a punch-drunk boxer.

For the first time in my adult life — I was experiencing the power of self esteem.

****

By the middle of September, '67 we were on the road again.

Checkpoint One-Four, the small log bridge was just ahead.

But this day something looked different; some kind of road work seemed to be taking place. As the driver coasted toward a stop twenty yards or so from the bridge, I noticed several pyramid-shaped piles of gravel being passed to our left.

With all the explosions that were taking place here, it had become standard procedure to have the combat engineers come forward and perform a sweep.

This day was no different. Following an innate instinct, the engineers waved their mine-sweepers at each of the piles. One of them signaled that he detected something.

On closer examination they discovered a hastily-camouflaged wire leading from one of the piles to a point under the bridge. One of the engineers cut the wire and signaled an all clear. Another probed the remaining piles and found that two of them contained precisely positioned Russian or Chinese made rockets ready to blast the crap out of us at point-blank range.

"OK. Good. They found them and no one got hurt."

Two weeks later, a Lieutenant fresh from stateside joined the battalion.

Most likely on the recommendation of one of his fellow officers, Sergeant M informed me that I had been requested to be his driver.

No big deal — just another new-guy wanting me to show him the ropes.

****

My first day with the new officer started like most: We traveled along Highway 1 towards Hue; the scenery the same as always: skinny dogs that seemed to belong to no one; old mama sans tottering along under loads of rice or shiny rectangular cans of water balanced on a wooden yoke. There were ARVN soldiers holding hands in the typical Asian way of showing friendship with other ARVN soldiers; giant water buffalos urged forward with brittle switches by tiny brown children. There were smoky little buses; barbed wire; children without legs or arms; children on crutches; the smell of fish and wood smoke; exquisite young women in white silk, gliding along on bicycles.

As we approached each checkpoint, the procedure required my response to my counterpart in the mine truck.

But at the first checkpoint, the Lieutenant grabbed the microphone to acknowledge him.

“Uh, Roger that Beach Boy Advance,” he said in a clumsy manner.

This is Actual — Uh, Out.”

I let it go — this time.

But as we neared the next checkpoint, I placed the handset in my lap, and as much as I knew it was a gamble, I told him in a respectful way that it was the battalion practice that radiomen did the communicating.

He grunted — seemed to be somewhat put-off by my insolence — but he relinquished.

By the time we reached Checkpoint One-Four; (14); the bridge — he still seemed uptight.

Maybe he was briefed that this was a hot-spot and he was nervous.

For some reason though, he must have felt that it was necessary to get closer, so obeying his instructions, I maneuvered the Jeep around the mine truck and took a position very near to the bridge where we both exited.

We were standing in front of the vehicle, waiting for the engineers to come forward and do their sweep and I recalled the rockets that had recently been discovered here.

We had been way too close that day — maybe as little as moments from being blown to smithereens. This day, I seemed particularly conscious of something bad unfolding, especially with the two of us standing in the open so obviously exposed.

My first feeling that something out of the ordinary was at work, was that on most occasions, after a few minutes of holding up traffic, several mini-buses would be lined-up on the opposite side of the bridge. Their passengers would be milling-about or chatting with fellow civilians traveling on foot.

But on this day, the road opposite the bridge was uncommonly empty and quiet.

So I had to wonder — did the locals know something bad might happen today?

Suddenly an old papa san, the color of tanned-leather from a lifetime of labor in the sun, emerged from under the bridge and ran along a shallow section of the stream.

He was dressed in nothing but a dirty loin cloth, and as he ran, he splashed in a flat-footed, distinctively sounding: PLOP! PLOP! PLOP! manner through the water.

In my mind, a mind bent on revenge, it was clear — he was nearly caught hiding a mine or detonator and was trying to escape.

I drew my .45; thumbed the safety to KILL (off), and led the old man like a hunter with game on the run.

I was a good shot and I held the front sight on the very tip of his nose. I was a millisecond — a thought — a blink from pulling the trigger and his head would explode. I had no thought of the consequences; no moral compass; no compassion for what I was about to do. I had decided in an instant that I was going to kill the old man, and that would be all there was to it.

The pressure increased on the trigger.

Then out of nowhere my wrist was struck.

I turned and snarled at the source.

It was the Lieutenant!

I knew better than to raise my voice or show disrespect to a superior and I said:

"Why did you do that, Sir?"

He was aghast and asked me what I thought I was doing.

Then he said something like:

“You just can’t shoot unarmed civilians!”

And he stomped off toward the Jeep and plopped himself down on the passenger seat.

****

We made it to Camp Evans without any further problems and while the trucks were being unloaded I visited a traveling PX.

I was thankful that things had moved so quickly. We would make it back to Phu Bai before nightfall. That evening, though I never heard it officially, I believe the Lieutenant reported me to the company commander for the attempted shooting of the old man.

That was fine with me! In fact, it was such a non-event that Sergeant M didn’t even bring it up.

A few days later I was back in the mine truck, and my new nemesis, the Lieutenant, was behind me, driven by one of the guys in my platoon.

In hindsight I should be thankful that at least one of us was thinking clearly that day at the bridge. When he stopped me from pulling the trigger he probably saved me from a "world of shit." For if I had killed the old man, I likely would have gotten a one-way ticket to the DaNang Brig or worse: LBJ: the infamous "tiger cage" Long Binh Jail: a sick acronym referring to the U.S. President at the time: Lyndon Baines Johnson.

****

By the first week of October, 1967, it was mild; slightly overcast, with temperatures in the 80's. All I would need was a short-sleeve shirt and my flak jacket. I had my helmet with me, but as usual I had it resting on the sandbags lining the floor of the cab.

As far as a weapon, I had recently been issued the second generation M-16; the one that didn't jamb as bad as the first one, and I had it resting against the seat with its barrel facing up and the stock nudged into a sandbag as well.

North of Hue, again approaching Checkpoint 14, my driver came to a stop at the usual spot just short of the bridge.

I don't remember what he did after he shut the engine down. Occasionally we'd stretch our legs or bum a smoke from someone down the line. More than likely he'd have done the same. I decided to stay put.

I was sitting in the truck; feeling relaxed; probably smoking a cigarette — why not — there were miniature packs with 3 or 4 smokes in each C-ration meal and a whole carton at our local or traveling PX was only two bucks.

Across the bridge, my attention was fixed on a fair-sized gathering of Vietnamese civilians waiting for the all-clear. Some were chatting with passengers through the windows of the three or four tiny buses which had lined up. On a small bank by the road, two or three old men squatted with their butts inches off the ground and their forearms resting on their bent knees as a chin rest.

As always there was the ubiquitous gathering of mama-sans, taking turns spitting blood-colored betel-nut juice from between their blackened teeth, while peasant women, old and not so old, urinated alongside the road through the oversized hems of dingy, paper thin black trousers.

With my right arm resting on the window frame, I could see in the long outside mirror beside me the images of the engineers walking alongside the column toward me.

There were three of them. One carried the mine sweeper. They'd do their thing and we'd be on our way.

In one corner of the mirror I could make-out the reflection of the convoy commander; the complainant Lieutenant. He was sitting in the Jeep, a couple vehicle-lengths behind me.

When the engineers were nearly beside me, I glanced again toward the commander's Jeep. I considered that I should contact the driver and repeat the incident about the rockets that were recently found here. With that, the officer would hear the warning through the speaker second-hand, and I would be vindicated, knowing that I had passed-on the message.

But by applying a little pressure on the mirror with one finger, I could see that the C.O.'s radioman wasn't sitting behind the wheel. For me to proceed with the warning would mean that I would have to speak to the officer directly — and I just didn't want to do that.

"Let him figure it out," I thought: "I ain't gonna help him be no hero.

That trivial criticism was my final memory of a world that until that very moment had made some semblance of sense as a wave of hot air swept over my right elbow. The surge was followed with a sound so earth-shaking — so earth shattering, that it seemed as if God had shredded the very atmosphere around me as fiercely as if it were tissue paper.

At that moment, it seemed as if all the snapshots that defined my young life — the hurt; the terror; the letdown; the guilt; Parris Island; Sgt. M's lessons; the strange new self-esteem; the Marine code to keep surviving above all costs, were surging within-and-without-me like magma.

And then, much like the day I was struck from behind while riding my bicycle, I was lying in a swale beside the road. The grass was dry and prickly, just like it was that morning five years earlier.

A humming sound filled the air, like a loudspeaker fading in-and-out. I believed at that moment that the end was near. I drew my knees tightly toward my chest to a fetal position and cradled my face with both hands tightly pressed against my eyelids and forehead.

In my mind there was no doubt — the NVA had an artillery piece zeroed-in on us and this first explosion was their adjustment round. The next shell would come in an instant, and with all that God may witness, I knew that I would then die.

Strange why it seemed to matter — as if somehow it might hurt less or be less ugly, but I pulled myself in even-tighter, waiting for the round to hit — exposing my backside so I wouldn't be vaporized from the front — praying it would kill me fast.

But the second blast waivered.

TICK-TOCK----TICK-TOCK

I imagined the cruel game I had read about, where North Korean soldiers during the terrible conflict of the 1950's, taunted American POW's in an execution ruse. The torture was carried out by putting an unloaded gun to a captive's head and pulling the trigger.

CLICK!

Ha-Ha. And they'd have a good laugh as the captured soldiers broke into tears having seen the face of death, and some went mad.

CLICK!

But I wasn't dead! --- I was alive!

Instinctively I ran my hand across and down my stomach, fearful of this worst of wounds, and then I checked my leg. Relieved, yet surprised to find no apparent wounds or bleeding, the words of my instructors at radio school then screamed to me:

"They'll all be depending on you to save them!" the voice said.
It was true — Time to get to work!

I rolled to my left side and sensing the familiar feel of my radio pack but not quite sure how it got there, I reached over my shoulder with my right hand and ran the pre-set dials to 39.50 — 39 point Five-Zero — the MEDEVAC frequency — the numbers burned forever into my memory.

Hearing the frequency come alive in the handset I shifted it to my right hand and extended my left outward to brace myself to stand. I knew immediately from the unmistakable suppleness of a human form that my palm was resting on a body; the chest of a fallen Marine to be exact, lying on his back beside me.

His buddy was bent on both knees beside him, supporting his friend's head with his forearm.

Pulling myself forward, I peered directly into the wounded Marine's upper arm. A precise hole had been punched through his bicep as perfect and circular as a machine that stamps-out auto parts.

Beneath the hole in his arm a divot of green grass was visible. No bone — no muscle — no blood; Just grass.

I looked up. The carnage encircled me like a scene from a horror movie and as my hearing returned, the air filled with the mournful cries of wounded and dying Marines.

Nearest to me, our Corpsman was treating a wounded Marine who was on his back not breathing. "Doc" had a plastic device held tight to the wounded kid's mouth and nose and he exhaled large breaths into it. I moved to his side and rested on both knees beside them.

Suddenly between breaths, the lifeless figure lurched upward, and with a deep, desperate gulp of air and bugged eyes as if he had been delivered from hell — he was back.

I asked Doc where he thought a good place for an LZ, a landing zone would be, and we agreed on a flat clearing near the stream. My primary responsibility was to contact the nearest medical unit and direct them to the LZ when they were in sight. But given the number of injured and seeing that Doc would have his hands full, I surveyed the scene for those who could be stabilized.

The inhumanity of the injuries of the dead and dying were staggering: One of the first dead I came across had been decapitated and the expression on his face seemed to give the impression that the head was still living; aware of what had just happened. The head seemed to be looking at its own body a few yards away and it was thinking:

"That can't be me — I'm right here — That poor guy over there got his head blown off."

Near the startled head, so close that if he had a foot he could have kicked it, a wounded Marine was sitting on a log, or maybe a stump, holding his severed foot with both hands. The Marine didn't speak to me, though it seemed he could have if he wanted to. But I could tell by the expression on his face that he seemed to be asking himself the question: "Where did the end of my boot and my toes go?"

About five yards from the toeless man was another body. It was burnt to a crisp. Both the burnt man's legs and arms were black and pink and red; blistered like charred salmon. His arms were frozen upward toward heaven as if he were calling the angels to take him home.

As I got closer, I discovered the burnt Marine to be a well-liked driver whose nickname was Pappy, even though he wasn't much older than his forties. Pappy had served with the Marines in Korea and reenlisted to serve in Nam. Some said his son was in the Air Force stationed somewhere near DaNang.

Near Pappy's smoking body, several Marines were standing in a semi-circle — hypnotized by the horror and at a loss what to do.

This scene of cruelty and tortured witnesses grieved me so badly that I felt that I had to eliminate it; not only for Pappy's dignity, but for those in pain at the sight of their friend, me included, his last day on earth, smoldering under black waves of burning tires.

I knew there would be a full can of water strapped to the rear of the lead Jeep, so I figured if I poured water on Pappy's body he'd stop smoking and I could cover him with something.

Purely out of courtesy, as now I guess I was seeing us all as victims, I thought I'd inform the CO (the Lieutenant) of my intentions.

"Sir, I said, standing close enough that I could have touched him.

I'd like to pour some water on Pappy."

But the Lieutenant didn't answer. He just stared straight ahead — paralyzed — unable to speak — both hands folded neatly atop his lap where his canvas map-case rested.

He had succumbed to combat's most contemplated question:

"Will I freeze when the shit hits the fan?"

Whatever contempt I held for him had disintegrated.

In fact, I felt bad for him;

I believe I even pitied him.

After all, I was still going and he wasn't.

As I carried the water canister toward Pappy, the sounds of Marines calling for God or their mothers filled the air.

I poured the water over Pappy's body until his Old Corps herringbone fatigues stopped smoking and I spread a piece of canvas over him.

In the distance, the first MEDEVAC appeared like a dull dragonfly zooming parallel with the horizon.

I walked to the stream and threw a canister of smoke to mark the LZ and establish contact with the pilot.

"Any med station this is Beach Boy — Over," I said, with the pure confidence of a seasoned vet.

"Go ahead Beach Boy," the chopper pilot replied, with a voice clattered by vibration.

"This is Beach Boy — Do you see my smoke," I said.

"This is Delta Med, Beach Boy. I see your yellow smoke."

"That's affirmative," I said, and I held both arms upward as a final signal to land.

Doc was supervising the transfer of wounded to the LZ as I walked back to the Jeep with the empty water canister. More wounded were lying here-and-there among the vehicles and as I made my way along the column, a Marine with no legs, only shredded rags where they had been, was calling for his mother to help him:

"Help me Mom! — Help me!" he cried.

Another called for God to help him!

"Help me God! — Help me!" he cried.

Reeling under the cruelty of their injuries and my increasing despair with their pleas for help, I was suddenly struck with an unashamed clarity: Despite the sounds; the smells; the tortured souls; the odor of blood in the air — Suddenly it was clear!

I was doing it!

While dozens around me were in a daze, or frozen, or vomiting, or rambling in circles — I was doing it!

I could feel the power of personal worth coursing through me as I walked from the LZ back to the road. Along with it, a voice seemed to surface within me; reassuring me; praising me. But then my world-view-reality seemed to sputter, like the spastic slow-motion wobbling of dancers in a strobe-lit discotheque.

As I neared the middle of the road, I saw a disabled Ontos: a small tracked-vehicle with three 106mm cannons mounted on each side.

I could see from the distinctive green clothing and somewhat human features that a body was slung-over the topmost barrel.

"Hey, help me get him down," a voice called from above me.

The strange inner-voice reassured me.

"[Sure, I'll help]" the voice whispered.

And on it went:

“[I’m handling it — See]”

Yes, I see

“[I’m handling it]!”

“[I’m doing it]!”

Yes, I see.

“[I’m the best radioman they got]!”

“[I’m going to save you — I have to — they told me I had to]!”

I’m ready — I can do it!

“Hey, help me get him down!” the voice repeated.

I turned and saw that the Marine calling for assistance was wrestling a limp, dead comrade off the barrel.

I reached out with both arms and prepared to receive the body of who most likely had been the Ontos’ operator. He would have been standing in the driver’s hatch — exposed, when the blast occurred.

I put my right arm under his neck as his upper body descended, and I braced myself for the expectation of a person’s full weight. Instead, as he flopped into my arms, it was as if a child had been delivered to me, as nothing but his bottom torso from the pelvis down rested in my left hand and the upper-half of his body wiggled its way onto my right hand. All that was connecting his two-halves together was his flesh-stripped spine — red and bumpy like a grotesque slinky-toy tapping lightly against my belt buckle.

He was young like all of us. His face was plastered with blue contusions from the blast which formed an eerie palette of dots in every pore.

I didn't know him: He was a fellow Marine — that's all that mattered.

He was someone's son; someone's friend — probably someone's true love.

I stared fixated at his disfigured face. Something was happening. Something was changing in me and I moved forward, still cradling the young Marine in my arms — still reeling.

Suddenly I experienced a frightening awareness of what crazy people feel like. The feeling was so real I felt that if I met another person who was mad he might say:

"Hello.... I know how you feel."

It scared the hell out of me! I thought that I was seconds away from going insane. North Vietnamese soldiers have documented the same reactions; of men going mad under the bombing of American B-52's; some putting pistols to their heads and blowing their brains out; Others walking in self-sacrifice into the furnace of napalm.

With the Marine and his two halves still cradled in my arms, I walked toward the side of the road, planning to lay him in the grass. Suddenly from my left a grunt Sergeant appeared.

He pointed directly at me and hollered:

“Don’t step off the road! — There might be another one!”

So I was standing at the edge of the road with this dead kid in my arms — my foot suspended in mid-air, as a second admonition shot through me:

“Oh God! What if there is?

What if someone stepped on something that detonated the first one?

What if I step on another one?” Then there will be even more deaths and horror and it will all be my fault!”

I never thought, nor did it matter, that I’d be dead too. What was more important to me than dying, was not to be at fault — to not be guilty.

“Oh no!” I thought. “Maybe this is already my fault!”

“Maybe if I had radioed the officer, this thing, this bomb, whatever it was, would have been found and none of this would have happened.”

I turned with the dead body still cradled in my arms and took slow, meticulous steps toward the opposite side of the road from where the Sergeant had shouted the warning.

A Marine who was standing in my path, looked at me, then at the disfigured body in my arms, and he bent with one hand on each knee and vomited in thick splats .

Passing the puddle of vomit I became more disoriented with each step. When I reached the opposite side of the road, I let the body slip from my arms where it folded at my feet in a macabre and twisted heap like a broken puppet.

Then looking toward the bridge, I could see Vietnamese civilians gathering-up pieces-and-parts of family members and fellow travelers, carefully and reverently stacking them in grotesque little pyramid-shaped piles.

Many of them, like many of us, were stumbling about dumbfounded and wailing. All the while the pile grew taller.

I had heard about the Vietnamese needing to bury their dead with all their parts. Evidently they believed their souls go to their version of heaven in the form in which their bodies are buried — no hand here — no hand there.

Then there he was — the same old man who a few weeks earlier had run from under the bridge and escaped being shot.

He was sitting in the grass at the edge of the road with both legs stretched-out in front of him. It was an unusual position for people who never sit but squat.

The old man seemed to be staring in shock toward the vast scrub-grass plain before him. At that very moment, there was no doubt to me that he was either involved in what happened or in some way complicit.

I decided to punish him.

I grabbed an M-16 — I'm not sure if it was mine, and I walked toward him. My right hand was gripping the tapered part of the stock just behind the trigger guard, and with my left I cradled the barrel-guard, near the front, just below the flash suppressor and sight. This stance allows a blow to your opponent like a boxer's right cross, stunning your enemy so you can follow-up with a bayonet slash to the throat.

As our eyes met I could see the fear in the old man's face. I closed on him. The red-rage of anger darkened. For a brief moment I could see terror in his eyes and he seemed to draw his body-in defensively, as if he'd try and take whatever it was that was coming.

When I was right on him, a figure emerged from some twenty yards away; someone who would be a witness; someone with the power to challenge me for what I was about to do.

But the red rage had grown more powerful with each step, and when I spotted the old man's metal cups and a smoke-stained teapot sitting next to him, I kicked the whole lot so hard that they rattled across the road.

At that instant everything went blank and a long time passed. There had been other times in my life when the red rage had overpowered me to the point of unawareness, like the morning my stepfather was beating my mother and I drug him off her and punched and punched him over and over in the groin until he collapsed. When I returned to reality, he was on his back with me on top of him. I had my left hand on his throat and with my right I held a tall teak statue of a Jamaican princess above his head, moments away from smashing his skull to kingdom come.

Those few moments near the old man felt the same.

Later, I don't know how long it was, I was on a barren hilltop at Camp Evans, walking toward a small portable water tank. As I got closer, a group of Marine grunts had gathered around it and were staring at me.

I was covered with blood from my waist to my knees and up both arms to my elbows.

I waved my forearms under the tap and watched the blood run over my hands and through my fingers, disappearing into the wet sand below me.

Hours or maybe days later — I'm not sure — we arrived back in Phu Bai.

I remember that I helped unload something resembling a dump truck once all the vehicles were back in the compound. There were a lot of bodies in the back and one at a time a Marine standing among them in the bed would pull one forward, where those of us manning the rear would load it into a field ambulance.

The last one I grabbed didn't have any legs, and it seemed like he was looking at me, asking me to hurry so he might be OK.

Is that possible?

I don't think so.

That seems impossible.

But I think I tried to prepare him for the inevitable:

"Damn man — you don't have a chance," I said.

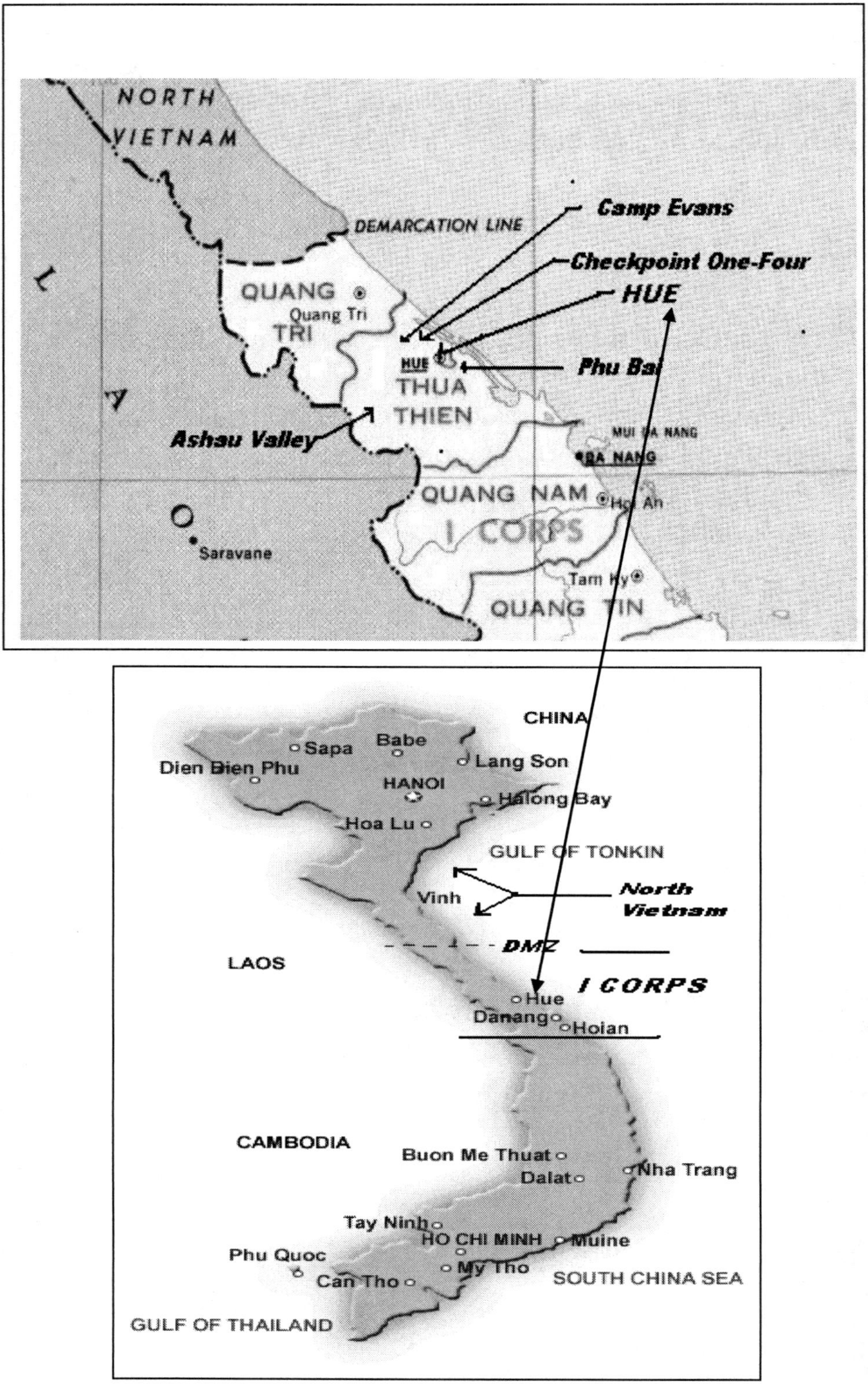
NORTH VIETNAM
DEMARCATION LINE
Camp Evans
Checkpoint One-Four
HUE
QUANG TRI
Quang Tri
HUE
THUA THIEN
Phu Bai
Ashau Valley
MUI DA NANG
DA NANG
QUANG NAM
Hoi An
I CORPS
Saravane
Tam Ky
QUANG TIN
CHINA
Sapa
Babe
Dien Bien Phu
Lang Son
HANOI
Halong Bay
Hoa Lu
GULF OF TONKIN
Vinh
North Vietnam
DMZ
LAOS
I CORPS
Hue
Danang
Hoian
CAMBODIA
Buon Me Thuat
Nha Trang
Dalat
Tay Ninh
HO CHI MINH
Muine
Phu Quoc
My Tho
Can Tho
SOUTH CHINA SEA
GULF OF THAILAND

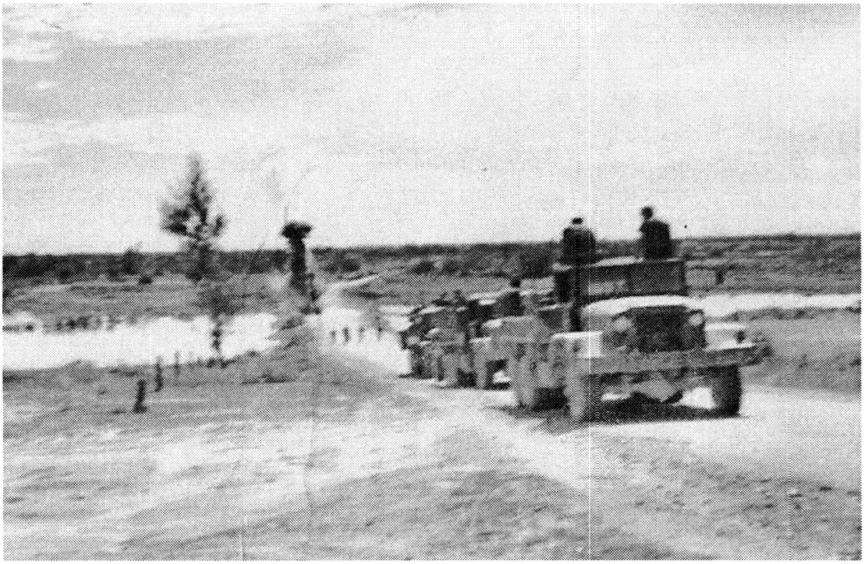

The actual Checkpoint One-Four is the bridge where the mushroom cloud is rising. On this day, Combat Engineers (the four figures at bottom of hill) found a road mine which they detonated. Less than two months after this photo was taken, an enormous blast killed dozens of Marines. By then, the large tree to the left of the explosion had been removed and the clearing was used by the author and a Navy Corpsman to land rescue helicopters.

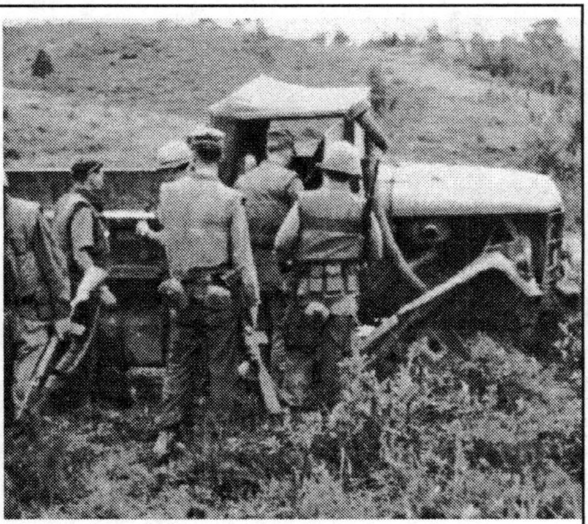

Early in 1967, road mines mostly disrupted convoys (like pictured) and caused collateral injuries to personnel. But by mid-summer the introduction of heavy explosives were causing us to have devastating destruction and deaths.

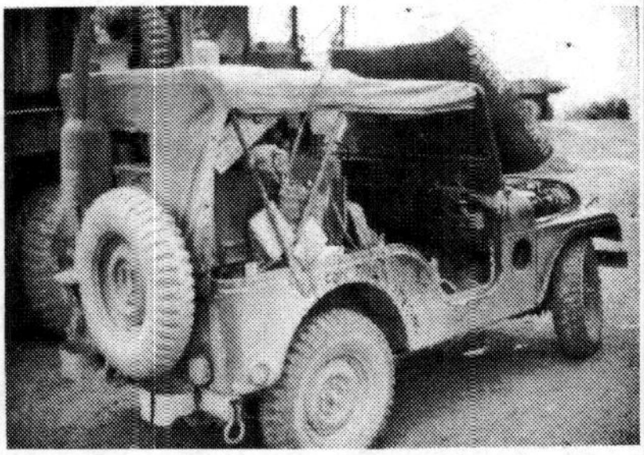

MRC-83 radio Jeep used by the author's platoon as a rear-guard vehicle during extended convoys. A message scribbled in the rear fender's mud says this convoy is on its way to Con Thien, near the DMZ, where Marines of the 9th Marine Regiment were about to engage in hand-to-hand combat with North Vietnamese soldiers.

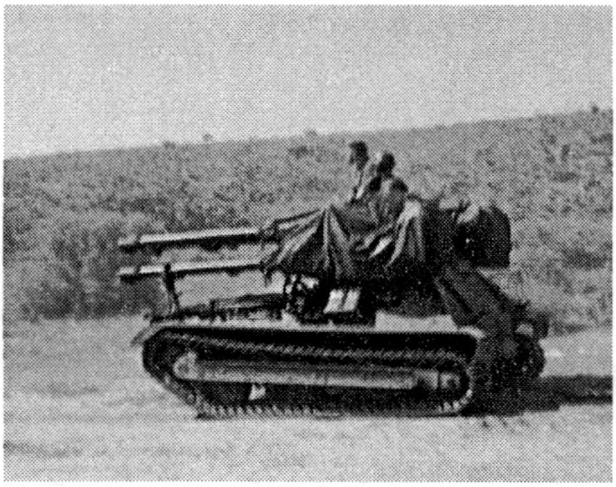

An Ontos like this was on the author's convoy when it was ambushed by a 250 # explosive device; most likely a rogue U.S. bomb retooled by local V.C. On that occasion, the vehicle's operator (pictured in the rendering below) was killed.

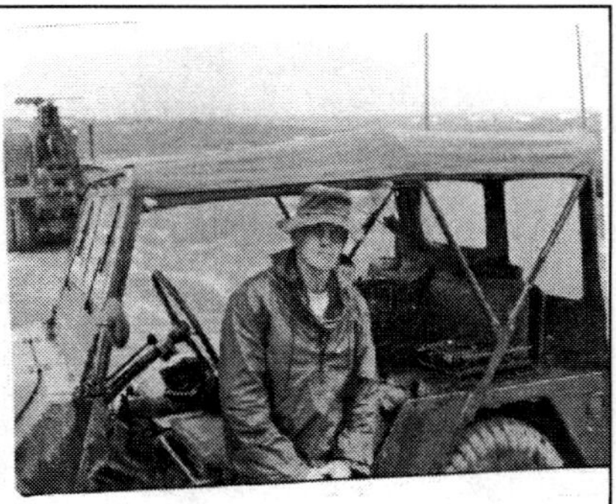

The author at the Marine combat base at Dong Ha, just south of the DMZ during the monsoon season of 1967-'68.

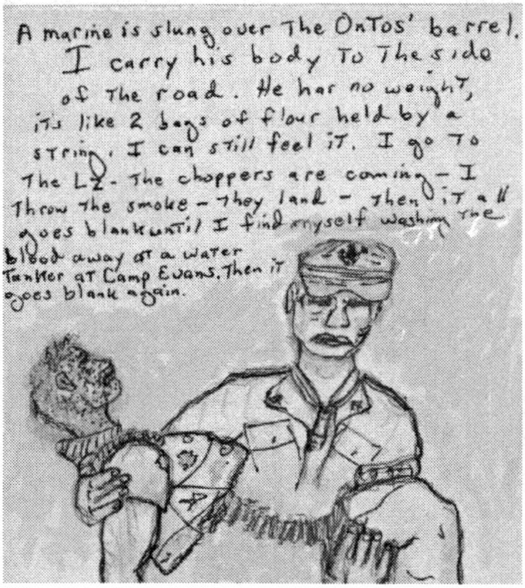

My counselor called this a "therapeutic drawing." Among the half-dozen I drew of my event, this depicts the scene I have lived with each day since 1967.

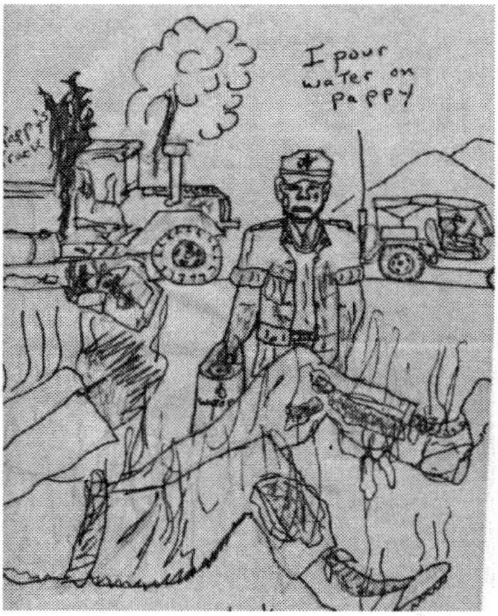

In this drawing I show myself carrying a water container to pour on "Pappy" who was blown from the vehicle shown in the background. My counselor found it interesting that I made a point of depicting the officer frozen in his Jeep behind me.

IV

SNAP

There is little doubt that the 1968 Tet Offensive (January-February) in South Vietnam was the tipping point for President Lyndon Johnson's announcement to the nation in March:

"*...With America's sons in the fields far away, with America's future under challenge right here at home, with our hopes and the world's hopes for peace in the balance every day, I do not believe that I should devote an hour or a day of my time to any personal partisan causes or to any duties other than the awesome duties of this office--the Presidency of your country. Accordingly, I shall not seek, and I will not accept, the nomination of my party for another term as your President."*— Lyndon Baines Johnson

Eight years into the war, nearly every household in America was touched in one way or another. By the time of the President's declaration in March 1968, nearly 1,000 young men were dying each and every month.

Vital to the advance of America's war machine, my battalion began moving north to Quang Tri, where an airstrip capable of accommodating the massive amounts of men and equipment needed in I Corps was nearing completion.

Just a few days before the first of March, 1968, our platoon sergeant: Sgt. Morello, rotated home. I hated to see him go, but I was especially bothered that prior to leaving he had put a "new guy" in charge of the platoon. The new arrival had the rare opportunity of arriving in-country as a Corporal — an E4. This fortunate act of timing for the new guy didn't give Sgt. M much choice I guess. None of us were any higher in rank than Lance Corporals — an E3, making this windbag with an annoying demeanor and nasally accent like a New York cabbie, the senior enlisted man.

I guess Sgt. M knew I disliked the cabbie Corporal, so as a final act of recompense, he ordered me and my close friend Joe C to catch the next convoy to Quang Tri. Our mission was to begin establishing our battalion's future communications.

Only a few days had passed prior to Joe and me heading north, that the 1st and 5th Marine Regiment had pushed NVA (North Vietnamese Army) soldiers across the Perfume River. Soon after, Marines stormed and destroyed the last of those fighting to the death from inside the ancient Imperial Palace: The Citadel.

In a scene reminiscent of the flag-raising on Iwo Jima, a Marine fire-team scaled a mountain of rubble within the palace walls where one removed an American flag from under his flak jacket and tied it to a makeshift pole.

As "Old Glory" punched through the haze that February morning, cheers echoed from every corner of the city as battle-weary Marines from trenches and rooftops, let loose a thunderous, unified roar for their fellow Leathernecks.

They had won!

As my friend and I made our way through the city, I marveled at the faces of the young Marines, who under horrendous house-to-house combat, machine gun and mortar fire, engaged and killed more than one thousand, battle-hardened soldiers. These young men would not realize for decades, that they'd be hailed among the legendary warriors of Marine Corps history.

Further on, at the approach of what was once the massive Checkpoint 26 bridge, I was shocked by the sight of its twisted framework; bowed and broken like the back of a slain beast, swamped in the river rift, courtesy of a U.S. Navy UDT (Underwater Demolition Team; later Navy SEALS).

Everything I had witnessed on a nearly daily basis while traveling through the city was destroyed: All the shops that had once lined both sides of the streets had been burnt to the ground or ransacked. In a bizarre scene only possible in war, the column paused as Marines armed with automatic weapons and grenade launchers zoomed through intersections in '60's-era Chevy Belairs.

Other stuff went on — some were rumors — some I saw. But one thing is certain: whatever the Marines did at Hue was nothing compared to the sacrilege leveled on civilians in the early hours during the NVA takeover. A short hike west of the city, even hardened troops were struck silent at the sight of the mass graves. From afar, the burial site resembled winter corn fields back home, where all that remained of the harvest were ragged russet stalks.

But up close, there was a sudden, gut-wrenching revelation. It seemed obvious. Many of the dead — women as well as children, had been buried alive, as witnessed by the zig-zagging rows of arms and hands of every size pleading from beneath the sand.

Back on the open road it was damp and dismal, yet a relief from the sights and foul smells of the city. And though hungry and cold, Joe and I arrived at Quang Tri several hours later in fairly good spirits.

For nearly a month he and I had it made: There was a makeshift chow-hall serving warm food nearly every day and hooches had been built so we were out of the rain.

There was even a one-man shower made from pallets, probably built by Navy Seabees for their own use during construction.

Atop the shower was mounted a cigar-shaped wing tank, probably from an old fighter jet. A rectangular opening had been cut in the top of the tank to accommodate a kerosene heater, like those we'd submerge in a garbage can for sanitizing mess trays.

This was beautiful! The opportunity for two Lance Corporals to control their everyday activities was too sweet to be jeopardized — so we hatched a plan.

We knew that eventually some uptight officer or Gunnery Sergeant sensing our lax regime would surely throw some stupid make-work assignments our way. So as soon as we organized our gear, we assembled the portable antenna we had brought from Phu Bai. Joe even attached phony *HIGH VOLTAGE* notices to the guide lines, which immediately caused people to give it a wide berth.

This particular antenna, a 292-something, was at best mediocre in performance, but its conspicuous height gave passersby the impression that it meant business. Enough so, that we were able to convince the acting C.O. that we were conducting relays for a radio group further north. And it worked!

By the time the other members of our platoon arrived from Phu Bai, I was less than thirty-days away from rotating home, and Sgt M's replacement; "the cabbie," more or less let me do whatever I wanted each day. I sealed the deal one afternoon in a boxing match where I destroyed a tall black guy from an Engineer Battalion.

I believe the cabbie corporal and two of his suck-butt buddies had me pegged as less than the street fighter I appeared to be, so when the challenge went out for someone to fight the engineer, I think the trio thought I'd lose, or that I'd chicken-out. The result was the engineer conceding after I knocked him down for the second time.

An April morning shortly after, just days from my expected departure date, the battalion clerk called me by name as I walked through the compound. He was a large Latino named Angel. He said that my orders had arrived to go home. That meant I'd be leaving five days earlier than counted on!

As I walked toward the mess tent, I felt like I was stumbling under the weight of the words.

Could it be possible?

Was I really going home?

"Hey Joe; Hey Paul; Hey Craig — I'm going home!

Yeah! — Really! — I'm going home!"

That evening I was still somewhat numb from the news. I made a canteen cup of instant coffee and sat on the steps of our hooch. The sunset was slipping behind the mountains toward Cambodia.

Between long exhales of smoke from one Marlboro after another I'm sure I prayed, in whatever way I prayed then, that nothing would go wrong before morning came and all this going home "stuff" was just some crude joke or mistake or nightmare.

"Please God — don't let anything go wrong."

Toward the top of the camp I could see my friend Joe's outline framed against the sunset. He was moving my way. Both his shoulders were pulled upward, as if he were trying to touch each ear with them at the same time. His arms dangled at his sides as if they were rubber. His neck was bent downward, as best as one can when trying to imitate a vulture, or bogey man, and he walked toward me with this weird, familiar, comical-look in his eyes like he often did, as if he were home in Indiana playing monster with the kid next door.

"Hey, Joe," I said, and I scooted aside to give him a seat beside me. There should have been mountains of words to say, yet my last night with my closest friend seemed awkward — I was leaving and he wasn't. What could I possibly say? And I recalled the many times during my thirteen months in Vietnam where I had been the one in Joe's seat, sitting next to someone leaving; wishing with all my heart that I was going with them, but knowing that that was not going to happen — knowing I would have to wait my turn: 395 days; 300 days; 297; 250 and so on, and so on, until all you can think about and all that mattered were the numbers — the slow, more important than anything, number of days left.

I slept well my last night in Nam, lulled to sleep by the familiar sounds of C-130's and choppers coming and going at the airstrip.

At morning chow I said my last farewells, some genuine; some not so much. I wrote the names and addresses of a few of the guys I considered my friends in a small blue pocket-sized notebook with Truong-something in gray etched on the cover. I even wrote down requests they had for a care package I promised to send when I got home — but I never did.

After chow, Joe drove me down the hill to the airstrip where I'd catch a plane to DaNang. From there I'd fly to Okinawa and home. And before I knew it, the plane was trembling and growling upward and Quang Tri and Joe had disappeared.

This time I could care-less if the crew-chief prowled back and forth — my moment had come. And yes, once in DaNang, new guys reporting-in looked at me with the same wonder that I had my first day in country.

And it felt good — real good!

Can you believe it! In a few hours we'd be landing on Okinawa, and just a few days more and I'll be home; sitting in my Mom's kitchen!

I'm going home!

We're getting on the plane!

It says Tiger Airlines in big bold letters on the side!

It's going to be okay! — It's really happening!

The door is closing! — The engines are at full throttle!

And as thousands of Marines before me had done, cheers filled the compartment as the wheels left the ground and Vietnam and the whole damn frightening, insane, wet, hot, deadly, guilt-provoking, bloody, killing, hate-filled, ridiculous experience was reduced in seconds to a small green turd on the landscape below us.

Up in the clouds, the flight to Okinawa was surreal. Stewardesses in mini-skirts with skin as flawless and smooth as Tiffany crystal made their way up and down the aisle serving soft drinks. There seemed to me to be an obvious intent to avoid leaning across those seated on the aisle. I think that was the first sign, subtle as it was, of what America's mindset of us had become.

For any aboard who failed to see the stewardess's trepidation, then moments after arriving on Okinawa there would be no doubt that we had been chasing a dream of an America that no longer existed.

Okinawa was never expected to be a memorable part of my journey home even if I did make it. But standing on the grinder, the parade field, the entire group was instructed to strip-down to our skivvies and toss our jungle gear: boots; everything we were wearing, into a pile in the center of a large human circle we had formed. The Corporal in charge of the formation said that our gear was going to be taken to the dump and burned.

It was April 6 or maybe the 7th, 1968.

Then the Corporal went over the procedures for what would happen next. As if apologizing, he began to describe the disturbing events occurring at home:

"On April 4," the Corporal said, "a man named Martin Luther King was killed in Memphis. He was a popular civil rights leader."

Civil rights? — Huh.

"There are riots all over the U.S.," he continued, "with things especially bad in Chicago, L.A. and Philadelphia, so anyone heading or changing planes there should be extra cautious."

Cautious! — About what?

Then he told us about Hippies: people we had heard of but had never seen who were beating-up servicemen in the airport bathrooms. He told of a little old lady who pulled a pistol from her purse and shot an Army guy in

San Francisco. Then the Corporal talked about bombings and murders and looting and whole cities being on fire.

"Bullshit! — That can't be true," I thought.

Then the bomb shell! The warning I have never forgotten:

"For any among you who wants to carry a weapon home for your own protection," he said, "here's the procedure."

Carry a weapon home?

And in a straightforward, matter-of-fact military manner, the Corporal stated the facts as if he were counting cadence.

"To carry a weapon on your person back to the United States, go to the Post Exchange and pick out the handgun you want. You will then be given a form that you will personally take to the base Provost Marshal. There is a 24-hour waiting period for purchasing handguns, so you will have to remain on the base for one extra day as your fellow Marines head for home. Following the 24-hour wait-period, you can pick up the signed form, whereas you can return to the PX and purchase the weapon."

And he continued:

"In the event you decide to purchase and carry a weapon stateside with you, (*on a commercial airliner for God's sake?)* the handgun must be kept in a separate pocket from the rounds, or from the loaded clip if it's a semi-automatic."

"Any questions?"

Whoa! This can't be!

But what if it is?

Well I sure as hell ain't gonna wait an extra 24 hours to go home.

Not when I'm this close!

Me either!

Or me!

"Hell no," others muttered.

So three of us: myself; a tall Puerto Rican from New York and an Italian from New Jersey made a pact: We would stick together; never leave each other alone, no matter what. And if necessary, we will fight to the death together.

Thankfully that never came to pass. But there were some tense moments in San Francisco Airport as the three of us walked past aisle after aisle of young people our age, sacked-out on the carpeted floors. We figured, correctly, they must be the Hippies we heard about.

Arriving in our transit areas we said good-bye and in a short period of time I was watching the world below me growing smaller and smaller once again.

After a few hours in flight I always looked forward to seeing the streets of Chicago passing below. It meant that I was about 45 minutes from Cleveland Hopkins. And sure enough, right on cue, I was walking through this newfangled tunnel from the plane to the terminal, where emanating from the nooks and crannies of the flexible passageway, the smell of engine plants and steel mills left little doubt that I had finally made it home.

I called my mother; collect (for those too young to know: calling collect meant that when the party answered, the operator would ask the person if they would accept the charges). As her phone rang and she answered yes to the operator, I had prepared myself to hear about the strange occurrences of riots-and-such going on. But I had trouble wrapping my mind around the reality of what she was actually saying.

She told me that Akron — my beloved Akron; the place I dreamed of for months-on-end, was under a "state of emergency."

"A state of what Mom?"

"Yeah, the Governor has declared Martial Law," she said. "There's been all kinds of trouble since that King guy got shot and there's riots and shootings and fires in Cleveland. The cops are worried it will spread to Akron

— There's already been a bunch of looting and stuff going on here."

She said that she would contact the Akron Police Department for permission to travel on the freeway and was sure that given the circumstances of a son returning home there would be no problem. I gave her the number of the pay phone and she said she'd call me back. In a short time it rang and she said she was on her way.

The forty minute ride home to Akron that morning is a blank, and so are many of the details of my first two nights at home. I do recall that I was fascinated with the variety of shows on the television. But I will never forget that for at least one of those first evenings I was unable to travel any further than her front porch, as there was a 9 PM curfew.

I called the girl who wrote me the Dear John letter a few months into my tour, and drove my mother's car to her house on the city's tough south side. It was only about four miles away, yet a world away socially and economically from the comfortable, middle class neighborhood of Firestone Park where we lived.

It was an especially sunny morning for April. From a half block away I could see her standing on the front porch. She seemed so young. Her shoulder length hair seemed more golden than I remembered glimmering like it did against the discolored siding and drab surroundings. The rows of rundown houses and dingy bars seemed to punctuate the fact that from the moment I pulled onto the cinder lot beside her house, I knew that there would be nothing more we would have in common. We spoke for a few minutes. I was surprised that the feelings we once had for each other were gone. But it was a relief to come to terms with the fact that the anger and hurt I expected to find if I ever saw her again was now buried forever.

A few days later a family friend and owner of a service station contacted me. A customer had a car for sale. It was a gorgeous 1965 Impala Super Sport; black, with black bucket seats; a floor shift and more chrome inside and out than I had ever seen.

I paid $1200 for the Impala from the money I had withdrawn from my pay each month. Most days I drove my black beauty around the city with nowhere to go, or no one to see. I went to my aunt and uncle's house in the country quite a bit, but my cousin had enlisted in the Navy and he was gone as well. That was also true for most of my friends and for all those who weren't drafted or were incognito, some in hiding or living an underground existence from government pursuers, tipped off by informants for reward money.

It was a lonely time, and nothing seemed to matter much anymore.

So I just drove around.

Following a 30 day leave I reported to the 2d Marine Regiment at Camp LeJeune, North Carolina. I had almost one-year-to-the-day left on my three year enlistment, leaving enough time to deploy for six months to the Mediterranean living on a troop ship with the Fleet Marine Force.

Just days before shipping-out I tried to make it home on a two day pass, and in the moments following a downpour, I plowed my beloved Super Sport into the back-end of a tractor-trailer on the Pennsylvania Turnpike.

The official medical report from the hospital in Everett, PA reads: *Brain concussion and chest contusion*. I guess the contusion took place when the steering wheel hit me and the dashboard caved-in, pinning me to the driver's seat. Thank God, two unfortunate hitchhikers; one a sailor and the other who I believe was a Marine- recruit going AWOL, survived, but they looked pretty bad.

During my stay I was allowed to see them. The sailor had a massive laceration from front to back of his skull from where he flew over me from the back seat and crashed through the windshield.

And the Marine?

He motioned for me to come closer. I bent near him and he whispered: "I'm gonna use this to get out."
From the way he said it, I figured he meant he was going to use the accident to get out of the Marines.

My mother bless her heart, drove the three and one half hours to Pennsylvania to retrieve me. With no choice but to face the consequences, I rode with her back to Akron where I would fly to North Carolina and face my punishment.

The company commander: Captain Franzia, was a good guy, and the afternoon of the day I reported-back to LeJeune he summoned me to his office. The enquiry I faced is called Captain's Mass; a disciplinary proceeding less harsh than a court martial, but with serious consequences available when necessitated.

Standing at attention in his office I offered-up a Polaroid photograph of my wrecked car taken by my mother at the junkyard in PA prior to heading home. Captain Franzia took the photo and after a moment of contemplation he said that I had probably been punished enough — and that was it.

The next day he spoke at our company formation and without using my name he told my story, reiterating the consequences of going out-of-bounds on a two day pass and how easy it is to fall asleep at the wheel: a phenomenon called Highway Hypnosis.

It was July, 1968, just days away from my battalion of the 3d Marines, along with tanks and amtracs and an aircraft carrier would leave Morehead City, North Carolina. We would replace the fleet preceding us at the very hour we entered and they passed the Rock of Gibraltar.

I was proud to be assigned at 3/2 to Major Tim Geraghty's, Forward Air Control Team. I think the Major was amused by the correlation of our surnames: McGarrity meaning in Irish: (The Son) of Garrity; Garrity spelled in its Gaelic form: Geraghty.

Years after I served with him when he had been promoted to Colonel, Timothy Geraghty commanded the Marine presence in Beirut, Lebanon in 1983. After moving his Amphibious Unit from the airport to a massive concrete building, a suicide-bomber drove a truck through a hail of bullets from Marine riflemen seconds before the runaway vehicle and dead driver crashed into the lobby and exploded.

The resulting blast killed over 200 of Geraghty's Marines and Navy Corpsmen. In his book: *Peacekeeper's at War:The Marine Officer Tells His Story*, he describes how investigators and forensic experts from the United States calculated the force of the explosion as: "…the largest non-nuclear detonation in recorded history."

While in the Mediterranean, our FAC team usually made our way, or was inserted into a concealed position on shore. From there we could direct F-4 Phantom jets on training and strafing-runs from the carrier.

While training Hellenic troops in Greece, our team spent a week living in an old Nazi bunker on a mountaintop, and near the end of the deployment, we dug-in on a barren hillside in the Dardenelles: the strait leading to the Black Sea and Russia.

Our landing team returned to Camp LeJeune in January 1969, and in April I was separated a few days shy of my exact discharge date of May 17. I was offered an opportunity to go to the FBI at Quantico, Virginia as a communication specialist, but my heart was set on going home to Akron and nothing on earth was going to interfere with that.

I had a fat insurance check from the wreck of my Impala and with the help of my uncle who worked at Chrysler and with his family discount I rolled off the lot in a shiny new red Dodge Charger.

Those first weeks home I spent a lot of time by myself, trying to understand what happened and where everyone I knew and grew- up with had gone. Only three years had passed, but I think I was most disturbed to realize that I had no job or any idea of what I'd do with my life.

People I graduated from high school with were nearly done with college! They'd be making good money, even though I didn't actually know what good money was or what the real scope of an education meant in terms of dollars.

With each passing day the anger grew. What was I? I was nothing but a working-class kid with a strong back. But hey, the economy was still bustling I guessed, so I figured that when the time came to get a job there should be no problem.

With the last of my mustering-out money dwindling, I roamed day after day from one end of the city to the other; back and forth, back and forth, looking for something that seemed to have no definition.

Even my old corner hangout where I cavorted with hoodlums and tried my best to be as tough as them was deserted. The doorway I stood "guard" from night after night, in the worst kind of freezing weather, held no reminder of my existence other than the jagged scratches with a church key, a beer can opener, than my nickname carved in the wall of the stucco vestibule.

One evening, feeling very lost, I parked across the street from my old hangout's row of mom and pop stores. I sat on the Charger's trunk at sunset eating a chocolate Skyscraper cone from the Isaly's Dairy store.

With both feet resting on the rear bumper I reminisced about the dairy store manager, a cantankerous older lady named Bertha who would chase us from the entrance with a broom.

But even she was gone.

The world I had loved held nothing but empty memories, and young people my age, looked and acted more like beings from another planet.

I was an outsider — We were outsiders!

Even adults, who I thought would at least admire us for our service, appeared as if they were ashamed or too disheartened to look us directly in the eye.

And the girls we dreamed of?

Are you kidding me!

"Girls smoke dope and say the "f" word!"

"Can you believe it? — Girls!"

"They don't seem to care what people think of them!"

To top it off, their boyfriends were these skinny-ass, ugly, long-haired hippies.

Can you believe it!

"Damn man! Not one of them looks like they could kick *anybody's* ass!"

The whole thing broke my heart.

So like many disillusioned veterans, I searched for those things that held some resemblance of my past, finding it in people like myself; people as mad at the world as I was — people ready for revenge on everything and everyone who dumped on us.

So throughout those first months of my first summer home, I did my best to turn the world upside down. I melted into the subculture of the 60's finding allies in the world of outlaw bikers and long- haired radicals.

I drank alcohol every day, cruising the rural back-roads of my childhood and city streets of my teenage years with a bottle of Boone's Farm or Ripple wine nestled between my legs. Sometimes I'd get pulled over by the cops, but I'd flash my still-fresh military ID and they'd let me go.

The net result of a lot of bad behavior culminated in the early hours near the end of summer, 1969. I had been home about six months. A close childhood friend: John M, had decided the same afternoon as me, three years earlier after a tough day on a construction site, that we were going to join-up instead of being drafted.

John M was a stocky Irishman, built like a longshoreman, who earned two field promotions for bravery and a Bronze Star at Con Thien in '67. I often wondered if he had been an officer if it would have been a Silver Star — maybe a Navy Cross; the next highest award to a Medal of Honor.

What else do you give to a twenty year old who saves his entire battalion?

During my friend's weekly down-cycles from drunkenness, when he was sober so-to-speak and reasonably lucid, he was a dedicated tradesman at Firestone Tire and Rubber, who even among his closest friends, rarely mentioned Vietnam, let alone his nagging secret. Not even me.

But aside from that, I did know what he had otherwise been through. On one occasion we met in the same camp in Nam and spent the night swapping swigs from a bottle of Jack Daniels, courtesy of mama-san at the stream-crossing. His arms were covered in sores from living in the bush above Khe Sanh and the more alcohol he drank the more they turned an even angrier red.

He went home several months before me and though I'm not quite sure of the details, he ended up shortly after his return home in a mental facility where he managed to scratch out a letter to me about some nonsensical issue of how the nurses try and trick him during smoking sessions. After he dried out a bit they released him.

Almost to the day after I got home, John M and I were inseparable.
But on many occasions when we went drinking, his behavior would turn ugly toward me like clockwork, and anyone else for that matter. He would slam the bar with his fist then wield false accusations toward those sitting nearby, eventually proclaiming in loud visceral tones: "I'm not afraid! — I can do it — I can do it!"

During my friend's outbursts I knew that in a few short minutes he'd be leaving — off to some hole-in-the-wall beer-joint in a dingy part of the city where serious drinkers twice his age could get wasted without being bothered with petty conversations about wives or kids or how work was going.

I was too young to understand the reality of alcoholism, and too unaware of how badly so many of us had been changed by the war. But one thing was clear: something deep, dark and demented was haunting my friend, and it wasn't until years later, when he finally hit rock- bottom and was living in his car behind a biker bar, that he told me about an execution plan conspired against a superior by his platoon-members, when his battalion of the Ninth Marines was at Con Thien — living in a hell-hole of mud, barbed wire, NVA snipers and hand-to-hand combat.

Given that — drinking and acting in a bizarre, aggressive way didn't seem unusual. A typical night out would have John and I making the rounds of local bars and after-hours joints.

One particular night I had taken several hits of "speed" (prescription diet pills). It was late and nearly closing time at bars with a 2:30 license when we came across these two guys on the south side that John seemed to know and who I had heard of, but that was the extent of it. At "last call" we each ordered a beer and in light conversation with our new acquaintances they said they were going to an after-hours place south of the city. They added that it was in an old farmhouse.

As we finished our drinks, the two joked about it being haunted and invited us to follow them. And we did. But with each passing mile, I grew more uncomfortable, especially as the city limits and our familiar stomping-grounds in South Akron disappeared far behind us.

My instinct regarding these two dirt-bags was right! Inside the farmhouse we paid for two overpriced beers and as usual, whenever John and I went out, one of us would get into a fight. It didn't take much; a bump; a look or a snide remark. And so this night it was his turn — some kind of racial implication toward a large black guy standing near an old fireplace who seemed to fancy himself a bouncer or something.

I was shuffling back and forth in what was probably the parlor fifty years earlier, keeping watch out a window at my car shining red and bright under a lone mercury lamp illuminating the driveway.

Suddenly I heard a commotion coming from the kitchen and I figured the inevitable was taking place. Sure enough, three men who appeared to be part of the crew running the place were shoulder to shoulder in a semi-circle, blocking my friend into a corner near the stove.

I entered the kitchen and growled: "What the hell's goin' on!"

Two of the three men blocking John's escape turned and faced-off with me from a few feet away. A somewhat smaller guy withdrew a pistol from his waistband and pointed it straight at my chest. I was in a rage and screamed a string of nasty names at him, and stupid or not, I snarled and told him that I was going to take his gun and shove it up his ass!

He seemed confused — sort of frozen and frightened at the same time.

Okay Jim, now what?

As quickly as he had produced it, the gun man made a clumsy, almost appealing gesture to pass the pistol to his well-dressed, somewhat tougher-looking counterpart standing next to him.

Just as his accomplice took the gun, I sensed a movement and heard a whishing sound in the darkness to my left. I ducked, just as a large fist slammed into the wall above my head. That's when all hell broke loose with punches flying from every angle.

John and I muscled our way down a skinny hallway through a flurry of blows and obscenities. At the end of the hallway we busted-through a rickety screen door which collapsed inward in odd geometric shapes like a smashed kite.

Like I said, something told me that this whole farmhouse thing didn't look good, so when we arrived, I parked my car purposely so I wouldn't get blocked-in if it became necessary to leave.

The gravel driveway from the road to the front door and back again was shaped like an inverted teardrop. I shifted the Charger into low and blowing sideways past the front door, the tires peppered the house and the first of those following us with a hail of stones. In their wake, the air choked with clouds of dust and burning rubber as I fishtailed onto the highway and headed for town.

Behind us on the dark highway headlights pierced the lingering smoke. An unknown number of people from the farmhouse were evidently pursuing us in a high-powered Chevelle. At one point the driver doused his headlights and passed us. Breaching an oncoming hill ahead of us he positioned his car sideways in the road to create a roadblock.

As I topped the hill I could see the bronze outline of the Chevelle turned perpendicular in the road. I shifted the Charger into low and with its engine rumbling, I rolled slowly toward them. In the headlights I could see two men standing outside the car. I coasted closer — revving the engine. Just yards from them I threw the wheel to the left; pushed the accelerator to the floor and kissing the Chevelle's front bumper and a wall of weeds, I whipped the wheel back toward the road opposite them and launched onto the highway.

We arrived at my mother's house seconds ahead of the Chevy and I ran into the house for my own pistol. John had already taken a stand at the top of the bank above her driveway.

As the two pursuers climbed the yard and were feet away from my friend I appeared. I held my pistol with my right hand, competition style, with the front sight pointed directly between the driver's eyes.

"Hold it!" I hollered, which stopped them dead and woke most of the neighbors.

Both he and his passenger raised their hands in surrender. With their arms held high, I backed them down the yard to their car and ordered them inside.

I was wild with anger, almost as angry as I was that day at the bridge. No sooner had they thrown themselves into the bucket seats than I was at the driver's window with the Luger poked firmly atop his ear. The safety was off — there was a round in the chamber and *Geladen:* German for loaded; visible in grey patina beside the toggle.

My mother never could keep out of things, and as I railed at the driver to throw his keys out the window, she danced back and forth between us in her nightgown.

Standing outside the passenger's window my friend was raging:

"Shoot him Jim!" "Shoot him!" he screamed. "Give me the gun, I'll do it!"

"No man! Please! The passenger pleaded. "Don't do it!"

My mother cried out: "Don't shoot him Jim! Shoot me if you have to kill someone!"

From the bedroom window next door, my mother's neighbors laid in the darkness taking it in.

"Do you think he will?" I later learned, the husband asked his wife.

My sister Diane, who was 8 years old, also watched the drama unfold from the living room window.

Once again — something or someone was watching over me.
Within minutes, several police cars were lined single-file in the street. In the bluish glow of a street lamp I saw two with their pistols drawn. Another was using the branch of a skinny tree near the curb to brace a shotgun.

As I decompressed emotionally and the red rage crumbled with police demands more desperate, I backed a short distance away from the Chevelle and raised the Luger in the air. With both hands held high, I ejected the magazine with my right thumb and it landed on the concrete with a distinct: CLUNK!

One officer took the weapon and cleared it, while another led me to a cruiser and the same for my friend. Since it appeared that all I had done, and the law dictated, was protect my mother's property, they confiscated the gun and let us go.

The next day I called a beat cop I knew from my days on the corner who was now a detective. I met him downtown where he wrote me a release for my pistol.

I was intrigued that he seemed to admire my service in Vietnam and asked what plans I had. I said I didn't know, and he suggested that I consider going somewhere like Los Angeles or D.C. and becoming a cop.

I didn't say it — but I thought it:

Are you kidding me! I was offered a free ride to the FBI and I turned it down. Why in the world would I want to be a cop in California?

But within weeks I was asking myself if I should have reconsidered, as the $1200 in savings bonds I had cashed-in and had lived on since returning home was gone.

I was broke!

One bright side of wars, if there is one, is for those able to or with the means or influence to avoid the draft, was lots of jobs. I learned quickly that many employers expressed concerns over hiring Vietnam vets, as we had already earned reputations for violence and drug use. Conversely, and I guess paradoxically, the deep-seeded disgust by another employer for anyone remotely resembling a "draft dodger"- type or so-called "hippie" with long hair and a beard — especially long hair, could work in our favor.

“Hey Alice,” blue collar guys would shout. “Get a haircut! “Yeah, or a flea collar!” another would chime.

So figuring that a strong back and still reasonably shorter hair than my contemporaries was still my best asset, I answered an ad for a laborer with a small construction company.

The owner and his brother interviewed me and I got a real sense right away that neither of them was impressed by my military service, probably because they had never served. But I was hired on the spot.

Three of us: Myself; Jack the foreman, and a forty-something likable black guy named Louie, made-up a crew building gas stations around Akron.

I liked the work, even though the owners were jerks, but the foreman was a fellow Marine who had served in Korea and we became friends from the very start.

Many construction workers went to a bar for lunch on Fridays; us included, where Jack would pound-down boiler-makers (a shot of whisky and a beer) and I’d try to impress him by keeping up. But most days I would get so drunk I couldn’t go back to work.
I quickly learned that trying to keep up with an “old school” bricklayer like him was impossible for a lightweight drinker like me.

One particular morning, Jack was late arriving at a jobsite near downtown. He had a notorious drinking problem like so many tradesmen back then, but I admit I was surprised when from atop a section of scaffolding I saw the company truck, a light blue Ford, careening down the street. Fortunately the traffic light had turned green just as he blasted through the intersection. Jumping the curb, Jack slid the Ford to a stop where a cloud of dust rolled over him.

"How do you dooo," he yodeled from the driver's seat, imitating the Johnny Cash ballad.

"My name is Sue — Now you're gonna die!"

Stupid me — I fell for it, and I leaped onto a mound of sand, where within feet of the driver's door I threw an amateur karate kick that caused a large, oil-can dimple to form right in the center.

Wouldn't you know it — moments afterward the owner's brother and financial partner, an uptight, all business jerk who should have concentrated on his dental practice instead of trying to be a construction mogul, pulled onto the lot.

As the dentist scratched his head; most certainly reflecting on how someone could possibly be so disrespectful, I confessed to him personally that it was my fault, and knowing it was the right thing to do, I told him that I'd be glad to pay for repairing it.

Evidently he decided that propriety meant more than recompense so he followed me to a large hole where we were preparing to pour concrete.
Peering down at me from the edge, the dentist announced in front of the crew that in addition to paying for the damage — I would have to apologize.

Apologize?

For what! — for a stupid little dent in a construction vehicle you arrogant ass!

I climbed out of the hole and looked down at Jack, who by the look on his face seemed to know what was coming.

The words just erupted:

“Screw you!” I said. And I got in my car and left, peeling off in a cloud of gray smoke and squealing tires.

Jack called me a day or so later to tell me that he had quit too and was going to Pennsylvania to work with a friend.

And that was that!

But dammit, now I needed a job again. It was nearing October.
Soon the snow would be flying and construction work would be harder if not impossible to find.

I never really thought that my military training would be useful in civilian life, but I had a knack for elaboration and got an interview as an alarm technician with A.D.T. (American District Telegraph).

The manager was an irascible old coot with a round red face and protruding belly. In his Navy days during WWII, it was probably what they called a barrel-chest until gravity and middle age sent it south. As he scooted in short bursts and creaking gyrations in an antique chair, I thought how he would have been just as at home in the front office of a muffler shop. There were stacks of small handwritten work orders scattered across the desk with an equal number impaled on nail pikes protruding from wallet-sized slats.

This was definitely one of those employers who hated hippies and appearing impressed that I had served in the war when so many were avoiding it, and with a modest electronic background in communications, he hired me at $2.95 an hour. The pay was lousy, even for the times, but I worked a lot of Saturdays at time-and-a half and we got paid for mileage.

I was doing alright.

I even moved into an apartment on the second floor of a rundown house not far from my mother's place. It wasn't much, but it was cheap; $55 a month and half utilities.

Then on a snowy night in November, I agreed to go on a double-date with the sister of a Nam vet I knew from high school. She was wearing a thick, fuzzy white coat, and she smelled like spring and summer all rolled into one.

We kissed in the back seat of her brother's car as we drove back to the city from a bar near Kent State. The window behind her was waxed with frost, and as the car flew through the frozen night, moonlight danced on her platinum blond hair, framed in a halo of softness from a silver faux fur collar.

She was tall by 60's standards — maybe five feet seven, with long, perfectly shaped legs that made her mini-skirts look like a handkerchief. Her name was Dorothy; a name she admitted not caring for very much, but I thought it fit her and from that very night, she became my true love and lifelong companion.

Dorothy was nineteen and I was twenty-three and throughout that winter and spring we spent magical nights cruising in the Charger and talking for hours at bars and dance clubs.

During the hours of conversation we shared very specific views of how couples should live as husband and wife and how parents should treat their children. We both came from families where upheaval was the norm and encouragement nearly nonexistent.

In Dorothy's case, even though her mother was a successful mid-level manager at a time when few mothers worked outside the home — girls, her mother believed, should plan on marriage and raising a family as a goal, and silliness, like wanting to be a flight attendant: a stewardess, as Dorothy aspired to and her mother discouraged, even after she was accepted as a candidate for a major airline — were unrealistic.

Obviously, that well-intentioned but frankly hurtful and outdated thinking influenced one of Dorothy's most powerful beliefs: that children should within reason, be encouraged to pursue whatever their interests might be.

As for my messages regarding success, my mother seemed insistent in pointing-out that success was something that *other* people achieved, and dreamers, like me, should be glad for what they've got. It was an odd ideal coming from a woman who endured daily ridicule and the systematic and brutal abuse of my stepfather.

Having spent many nights as a child listening to them argue and hearing her getting the crap knocked out of her, my promise to a relationship was simple — women should feel safe, loved and respected.

And men: Never! — Ever!! — Hurt them.

****

On a spring afternoon in 1970, Dorothy rode on the back of my motorcycle to a wooded metro-park south of the city. We climbed to the top of a hill overlooking a stream and a picnic area where I asked her to marry me. We toasted our engagement on the hillside with a bottle of Ripple and a small bag of potato chips. It seems a completely unromantic and derelict ceremony today, but then? It was cool! That's all that mattered.

Our wedding was a simple affair which took place a few months later in August. It was followed with a reception at the church, respecting her mother's wishes, and that night we held another to include alcohol in my mother's driveway with a makeshift bar set-up in the garage.

Before the wedding I realized that either the Charger or the motorcycle had to go, and believing that cars-were-cars, but my Harley was me, I sold the Charger for practically nothing and used the money to buy an ugly but fairly functional VW Karmann Ghia.

We managed to go on a modest honeymoon to Richmond, Virginia, even at the objections of my boss at ADT who threatened to fire me if I did. I did anyway.

A week later, Dorothy and I limped home on fouled spark plugs and just enough money to buy a tank of gas and two hot dogs each near Everett, Pennsylvania, oddly enough, near where I had nearly killed myself and two hitchhikers in a car accident two years earlier.

We moved into my second floor apartment behind a rundown and smelly Italian grocery store. The apartment wasn't anything to brag about, but we kept it clean; it had a private entrance and the use of the garage where I kept my motorcycle and where Dorothy and I spent many evenings; tinkering; polishing, and drinking coffee beside a little kerosene heater, talking about our future with the child she was carrying. Downstairs, an aged but friendly-in-a drunk-sort-of-way ex-barmaid and her adult daughter did their best to provide for themselves and the daughter's two wild children.

I've got room to talk! Dorothy, (affectionately nicknamed: Dort) and I became immersed in the wild and impulsive lifestyle of the '70's, with my friends being our friends — bikers and veterans and former high school hoodlums.

And Dorothy, who as a teenager had perfected her covert flights from the obedient daughter and Sunday school teacher from her parents, joined me in embracing the wild side.

Like she says — we were kids, having a ball and making-up for something neither of us would find easy to define — but admittedly felt damn good at the time, filling some overwhelming void, especially in me. Mostly, my angst came from the financial success my peers were poised for as mine was postponed due to war. And secondly, the destroyed self-esteem inflicted on me in ugliness that would fester for decades.

At least as the whacked-out biker veteran, I believed that I stood a chance against a world where disrespect, stares, and letdowns, tended to take a detour around me.

Thank God one of us was thinking clearly, as Dorothy almost certainly kept me from going to jail, or dying from depression, or assaulting neighbors, or crashing our cars in road rage incidents or a thousand other fits of idiocy toward a world where I believed, the only way to get respect came from hostility, or at least the appearance of it.

Somehow Dorothy knew that under the spell of the impulsive and suspicious Jim I created was the better person I really was — The child who in his early years, living in the country and traveling across America in an old Dodge bus with his grandparents, had a genuine sense of love and integrity and what doing the right thing was.

And with just a few words from her like: “You know — we have a daughter at home depending on us,” she could bring me back from absurdity.

Sensing it was indeed time to do the right thing, in 1971 we moved into a decent apartment complex in the city and shortly after I started night school at The University of Akron.

My plan was nothing sensational. I always liked analytical stuff and after reviewing a flyer from Akron

U's, Community and Technical College, I was intrigued with the possibilities of land surveying.

I qualified for free education under the G.I. Bill and was doing really well at Akron U. I was especially proud of the 4.0 grade in English and I even passed Math Analysis.

But even though I was a conscientious and often an enthusiastic worker who never missed a day and studied late into the night, there were occasions when the call-of-the-wild (and trouble saying no!) got the best of me; like the night I was studying for my final exam in Math II and gave-in to two so-called friends that stopped by.

What can I say — we got high on weed.

Later that night as I returned to the problems; man, I thought I was Einstein.

Unfortunately, the day of the exam everything was a blank. I didn't have a clue how to solve one problem. I had gone from Einstein to Alfred E. Neuman in a few puffs. As those around me labored away, I left the classroom and threw the crumpled-up test in the wastebasket as I passed through the door.

My instructor phoned me the next day and offered to work with me to make it up.

But I figured — why bother: "It's all B.S. anyway."

Thank God for my old friend Jack the bricklayer, who at the construction company three years earlier in 1969 had encouraged me to take an apprenticeship exam for the Plumbers and Steamfitters Union in Akron.

Just days after I walked out of Akron U, feeling very low and desperate, the letter arrived. It stated that I had been selected for an apprenticeship and that I would start work in two weeks. Standing in the simple surroundings of the apartment, with Dort in my arms, it seemed as if the weight of the world had been lifted from me. It was all I ever wanted! I was gonna be something! — making good money with benefits!

It was 1972.

Just in time! A new breed of tenants seemed to have arrived overnight, turning our apartment complex into a municipal housing disaster, where within a month, cops walked the night-beat with shotguns and parents stood guard at recess to keep bullies from attacking their children.

I had barely entered the first year of my apprenticeship when fortunately for us, a friend vacated a rented house east of the city and we took their place as its newest tenants.

Over the next four years, a second child Michael was born and Dorothy had become a full-fledged wife and mom who indulged much of my outrageous behavior and the image I had created for myself.

In 1977 I became a journeyman steamfitter and was making more money than any of our friends. It seemed that our life was actually on the right track.

Then in 1978, just a few days before Mother's Day, a lifetime of undiagnosed and untreated depression caught up with my mother and she shot herself in the stomach with a .38; an act that most experts say is contrary to how women usually kill themselves, being poison or pills.

It seemed she had always prepared me and my younger half-sister Diane for the inevitable, with morose comments about how a fortune teller had told her when she was a young girl that she'd die a violent death. Some evenings at the dinner table, our mother would gaze at the bridge spanning the freeway behind our house and say:

"I should just go over there and jump off."

But how the hell was I supposed to recognize that these were warning signs? And even if I had — who would I go to in those times to help her?

Like I said — It was just the way life was at our house.

After Mom's funeral, my sister Diane who was seventeen at the time and a senior in high school moved in with us.

Suddenly we needed more room.

I borrowed the money from my aunt and uncle for a down payment on a large home in the respectable, working-class neighborhood of Firestone Park, where Dorothy had grown up and I had lived since 8th Grade.

The three of us, Dort, Diane and I, were glad to be in "The Park" again, with its tree-lined, brick-paved boulevards; good schools and familiar faces. Within walking distance and overlooking the rambling tire plant he created rested the colossal bronze statue of Harvey Firestone, the holy-grail of coming-of-age ceremonies for "Park Kids" to discover the joy of sitting on "Harvey's" lap. A block from the house was a strip of old time stores connected like row-houses and providing many of our basic needs. Plus, Dort was within walking distance of her parent's house, where her closeness with her parents and younger brother had always existed, and time and an age-old conflict between her father and the oldest son had finally fizzled-out.

Externally our lives seemed to be going fairly well. But emotionally, after Mom's death and an accusation by one of her sisters that if I had been a better son it might not have happened, I began to believe on a grander scale that the world was more dangerous than ever; more deceitful than ever and definitely more unfair and hurtful than ever.

Coupled with the guilt surrounding mom's death and the shocking memory and images every single day, that if I had spoke up at the bridge that morning in Vietnam, the explosion might not have happened and all those guys would have lived, further stripped me of my capacity for trust and safety.

And even though I hadn't used narcotics in almost five years, I was still hanging with bikers I considered my friends, and occasionally I'd push the limits just far enough to keep respect, but not so far as to risk being pulled into the real troubles they involved themselves in.

What I failed to see was that the friends we had early-on in our marriage had moved-on and were succeeding with their lives. I on the other hand, had been pulled ever-inward into a circle of more violent and derelict people.

One day, a person I considered a friend and was a regular visitor at our house, stopped by unexpectedly. He and I were sitting on our front porch. I was waiting for an old friend, maybe the last real friend I had, who would be arriving soon with his wife and two daughters. As they exited the car, I was shocked by the quick and crude sexual comment the visitor made about the girls.

His words drove a stake in my heart. In a flash I realized that not only did I have a beautiful wife and a six year old daughter and baby son to protect, but I now had a teen sister who we considered a full member of our family. I was appalled. I saw only one thing to do — sever myself from my past and everyone and everything associated with it!

I was about thirty-one years old at the time.

From that day until I retired at age 55, I was the loner; the explosive guy; the target of plots guy.

I became the guy who never got a break.

I was the guy who could only watch from the sidelines as those I saw as less competent than me worked regularly, even though toward the end of my career in piping I received an award for craftsmanship.

But perfectionism on the job, as well as my personal life, had become an albatross, as striving for quality and safety turned to an obsession toward excellence, right down to the angle of the slot on a screw head.

And while renovating a hospital, the project where I was given an award from the Cleveland Builders' Exchange, I was blindsided by paranoia concerning germs, adding to an already-exhausting struggle with the laws of heavy mechanics and sudden death or injury.

As I wrestled to control my external world — my internal world was collapsing. Years of constant layoffs and financial struggles finally took their toll as depression drew me into its pit of hopelessness and shattered self-esteem.

Anxiety manifests in strange conflict with depression. You'd think that being down would be your hallmark but for me the opposite was true, as the further I sank the more desperate and hopeless rescue became. The first examples of this paradox came with horrendous panic attacks and the belief that I couldn't swallow unless food was chewed to mush.

Some nights I was frightened to fall asleep as each time I closed my eyes I saw the darkness with such black intensity that I panicked at going blind and would have to open them and wait for the night vision to come, reassuring myself it wasn't happening.

Other nights I would drive through the darkness of the interstates for miles, or occasionally, I would park on the moonlit dirt back roads of my youth, smoking cigarettes and listening to the familiar happier sounds of crickets and frogs and occasional barking dog.

But mostly, in the grip of winter and joblessness, I would slide down the wall beside the heat register and stare into space in the enormous living room or hope that Dorothy would take the children and go somewhere for the day — anywhere — so I could hide under a blanket; away from guilt and responsibility and mounting bills, unafraid of thoughts of falling asleep and not awakening.

But I knew the pain that seeking death can bring.

So I endured. And years passed.

****

In 1995, we got a cold-call from a real estate agent inquiring if we might consider selling our home, under the pretense that a young couple friendly with our neighbors loved our house and would we consider selling.

It was probably a sales strategy, but I had been working steady for a change, and we had actually been considering —well —mostly dreaming, about moving outside the city.

We signed a thirty day trial contract to see what we could get, albeit the mysterious, inquisitive house-hunting "friends" who never materialized.

We only owed about twenty thousand dollars on the house and were ecstatic when a couple from New York state came along; fell in love with it themselves and agreed to the full asking price of seventy-five thousand.

We found a small ranch house, 20 miles from the city in a tiny village of 3,000 and bought it on the spot.

Packing the giant steamship-of-a-house with its 20 years of accumulation was daunting, and I remember the evening I hauled two armloads of bound-up National Geographics to the curb (a task "baby boomers" consider nearly blasphemous) when a strange, suddenly-exhausting sensation washed over me.

"No big deal, we've just been working hard."

Denial?

You bet. My chest had been feeling strange since we signed the sales agreement.

Within a few days I had a heart attack!

It was a bad one!

Thank God I was working that day on a hospital renovation. It was a warm, humid morning and I had just finished throwing timbers back on the deck of a crane our crew was using. Suddenly I felt funny and was extremely hot. By the time I got to our work area my forehead was blistered with huge puddles of sweat. I sat on a stack of drywall to compose myself. Someone made a frantic motion to my foreman who took one look at me and immediately helped me toward a large plywood door separating the work area from the existing facility.

By the time he nudged open the door and we entered, I was unable to walk. I braced myself against the wall and slid toward the floor in slow motion when a nurse approached. She took one look at me, asked me my age and threw me into a wheelchair, racing through the hospital with one hand navigating us around startled visitors while calling “CODE BLUE!” into her handheld radio with the other.

I was unaware of the reality of what was happening, even with nurses gathered around me asking a thousand questions. But when the doctor asked if he should contact anyone, and I answered no, thinking I didn’t want to frighten her, it began to make sense when he quickly said: “I think we should.”

“You can call my wife Dorothy,” I mumbled.

This would be one of many close calls with death that Dorothy would face.

This day I was saved. The next day I was transferred to a larger facility where two plugged arteries were unblocked and stents installed.

Amazingly, a few weeks later I was back on the job. The guys looked-out for me when it came to the really hard physical stuff and soon I was back to my old self.

I was only 48, and Dorothy and I began a new chapter in our life — as country people — or at least people living in the country.

There were still the usual layoffs at work, but I didn’t seem to care anymore. I think I learned to not take the layoffs personally, as we had made it this far living on the edge and never in my wildest dreams in those early days on the second floor hovel behind Mr. Oriti’s smelly little grocery, could I begin to imagine us having anything like we had now, albeit modest and after 25 years together, still surviving week to week.

****

Years passed and America went to war for the second time with Iraq.

I admit that the 1990 liberation of Kuwait (Operation Desert Shield) by the United States, when Iraq's dictator Saddam Hussein invaded his small neighbor over oil rights, had become a secretive sore point for me as the public rallied around America's forces.

I was convinced that during the short period of the conflict, (Operation Desert Storm in 1991) the overwhelming outpour of patriotism was insincere, and all the yellow ribbons tied on old oak trees, as the hit song by Tony Orlando prescribed, and church-ladies' "goodie boxes" for the troops, were more about the guilt Americans harbored for not supporting Vietnam vets or, for avoiding military service themselves.

I wrote an editorial in the Akron Beacon Journal at the time with a veiled chiding directed at self-serving patriots who never served, nicknamed by some: Chickenhawks. Hidden in the words was a cryptic message pointing out that veterans of all eras deserve respect and recognition.

But for the most part it fell on deaf ears. I had done what I thought the phony patriots were doing, just in a different way: I was trying to make myself feel better.

Nearly eleven years later in 2002, America embarked again on a campaign to eliminate Saddam Hussein, based on President George W. Bush's belief and as far as I'm concerned, the king of the Chickenhawks: Vice President

Dick Cheney's fixation on Iraq's supposed nuclear weapons' stockpiles, popularized as WMD's, or Weapons of Mass Destruction.

Now I was really pissed-off.

As the death toll of U.S. troops skyrocketed, Bush reelection-operatives capitalized on the war by painting anyone with the slightest opposition as unpatriotic, combined with around-the- clock television ads discrediting the 2004 Democratic candidate, John Kerry's service in Vietnam.

As the daily drumbeat against Kerry persisted, I took it as a painful and personal assault on me and all veterans — especially Vietnam Veterans.

That's when the nightmares started.

It was sometime in September, 2004 when they got really bad.

I dreamed in shocking detail that I walked into a high school gymnasium where hundreds of wounded young men stood shoulder-to-shoulder on the main floor, staring like zombies toward the entranceway.

The bleachers on both sides of them were packed with wounded as well, all standing on the seats, waiting for me to sidestep down the rows where I was compelled to stop and assess each one for their degrees of injury.

That nightmare alternated with a similar theme, where I see myself walking into a troop-tent used as a morgue. There's an adjoining room, separated by a door with a small window.

A light from the other room beckons me and I move toward it for a closer look.

Through the clear plastic window I see that the floor in the small room is tamped-down dirt, with neat rows of brown folding chairs.

Each chair holds a wounded Marine, dressed in only his underwear and each is badly wounded.

There doesn't seem to be anyone paying attention to them.

Then one of the wounded Marines sees me peeking through the window. His face is dirty, like he'd emerged from a coal mine. His eyes seem to be asking me for help.

But there's nothing I can do.

The demons of Vietnam that had kept me locked in the belief that a mere radioman in a truck couldn't possibly be affected by war, had surfaced with a vengeance.

V

THE PROMISE

November, 2004.

Each day I sunk deeper into the clutches and clockwork of depression: angry – down – angry – down.

My existence became an ever-evolving web of mental endurance. Often, when Dorothy wasn't home and there was no need to smother the anger, I would stare at my reflection in the bathroom mirror and descend into rage — my irrelevance and helplessness mocking me; driving me to self-disdain and powerful open-handed blows on one cheek then the other — back and forth; cursing the face in the mirror for its living caricature of a "sad sack;" helpless to break free from the exact kind of person I despised.

Flushed and humiliated I would storm from the house, believing that all that was needed was to get moving — "Snap out of it!" — "Get over it!" — hoping, praying, that somewhere up the road or around the block something miraculous would take place; where the blanket of guilt and hopelessness would be lifted; A place where the ravenous emotions consuming me would turn to vapor.

But relief never came. By the time I reached the top of the hill or the first corner before the turn I would drown in-stride:

“Aw to hell with it — it’ll never change.” And I’d turn toward home in a slump — my chest hurting — my stomach boiling — my room calling me to draw the shades and escape: “… at least for a while please Lord,” from life’s demands and ultimate letdowns.

****

My mood was lifted when I learned that my daughter Kelly would be visiting us for a few days. Having her around always made me feel better. The first morning of her visit I was sitting in the kitchen, drinking coffee and watching TV as usual.

My daily struggle between misery and anger was its own vicious cycle, but mornings had become a special ritual-of-rage, driven by a swelling hatred for right-wing TV networks and Republican politicos belittling John Kerry, the Democratic candidate for President.

Kerry was a Vietnam veteran who served two tours in Nam, yet he was bombarded during the campaign by White House "chicken-hawks" (people who never served in the military but bang the drum for war) as a pinky-finger, east-coast elitist.

This was the last straw!

My anger toward these people became painfully personal and I wrote ranting diatribes by email to network talking-heads. Conversely, I sent messages of support to journalists and politicians who even hinted that their political persuasions and disgust for the Bush administration were the same as mine.

Unpredictable and runaway emotions weren't new to my children. My daughter Kelly and her brother Michael had grown-up surrounded by them. But as the wife of a rural minister and devoted mentor to young girls on surviving adolescence, Kelly had little patience with people who thrive on malice with so much good to live for.

Her first morning with us, she entered the kitchen as I was yelling at the television — pounding on the table with the usual diatribe of threats.

"Dad!" she said, admonishing me in a tone I had never heard before.

"Do you realize how bad it hurts me to see you so mad at the world?" And she disappeared toward her room.

Kelly's words hit me like a hammer. Throughout her childhood she saw me move from love to rage with the flick of a switch; with me the angry, unpredictable, yet conversely and fiercely devoted and protective father. And I believe that on some occasions, she and her younger brother felt empowered; perhaps emboldened by my reputation in the neighborhood as the crazy Vietnam vet on a Harley.

But on this morning, she had decided that enough-was-enough. She had made the decision that she would show me that she loved me so much, that she would no longer stand-by as I consumed myself with hatred.

"Oh my God! My precious child — my little girl hurts because ***I'm*** unhappy? What in the world can I do so she never has to say those words again?"

Stunned by her candor, I sat at the table reflecting on how the emotionally-charged weeks had affected me. But I had disconnected myself years earlier from the ability of self-reflection and the enviable human condition to comfort one-self; an aspect of intimacy, lost it is said, for people who are victimized.

But was I a victim? I thought that a victim was someone who'd been robbed or raped or murdered.

I happened to be going to the store for something-or-other and I asked her to ride along. On our way I told her about the frightening, war-themed nightmares I'd been having, and how badly depressed and angry I had been for such a long time.

I believed she could understand in some way. Kelly was extremely intelligent and unlike many of her peers, was aware, if not intellectually empathetic, of the troubles faced by Vietnam veterans like her father.

Incredibly, I was just days away from my first-ever appointment with the Veterans Administration. Seven years earlier, at age 48, I had a heart attack, and as the cost of medications skyrocketed and the deductibles on my private health insurance through my union's health plan soared, the monthly expenses were draining us.

All I hoped for and sought on this first-ever visit to the VA was some sort of help in obtaining the more costly meds. When I told my daughter about the appointment, she asked me to promise her that I would tell the VA doctor about everything I had confessed to her.

I agreed that I would.

A few days passed when I visited the VA Outpatient Clinic (Community Based Outpatient Clinic) in Akron. Following a swift but thorough physical by the VA Primary Care Physician, he asked if there was anything else he could do for me — or if there was anything I needed to talk about.

The night before, with the promise still as fresh as a wound, I had written-out the details of the nightmares, including some facts about one particularly nagging and troublesome incident that happened in Vietnam.

It wasn't the first time I had tried to face the facts of that day on paper. Many times over the years I had chain-smoked late into the night with pen to paper, trying to face the moment. Eventually, the result was to crumble-up and toss the twelve or thirteen or even twenty handwritten pages into the wastebasket:

"...who the hell would care what happened to me?"

So the morning of the physical I was completely in character when I hesitated to answer the doctor's final question.

It was a busy day, like most days for him must be I thought. It seemed like he was running behind so I figured, why bother him with a bunch of crap about nightmares.

I was moments from leaving the examination when I was struck by the promise.

"I told my family I'd tell you about this," I said, as I removed the folded sheets of paper from my hip pocket.

The doctor took the statement, leaned back in his chair and appeared to read every word.

In the letter I talked about the nightmares, and Vietnam, and what happened at a small bridge the day a lot of Marines were killed.

He read how I felt like I didn't care if I died, and that my chest hurt all the time, and how every morning since 1967 I've seen myself walking across the same road in Vietnam with "him" (I gave "him" special status with no explanation to offer) in my arms — so clearly — it was as if it happened the night before.

I appreciated how gently — how almost reverently the doctor laid the sheets of paper on his desk.

And then he looked directly at me and was quiet for a moment.

"I think you should talk to someone about this," the physician said. I'd like to schedule you for an evaluation with mental health."

The words caught me by surprise and I said:

"Because I've been down?" I said. "Couldn't it be that I'm just one of those people who are naturally sad?"

My question seemed to puzzle him but I think he already knew what the outcome would be.

"Let's let them decide," he said.

As I drove home that morning I felt oddly relieved. Many times during my years with Dorothy I wanted to talk to someone about the intense periods of sadness and anger. But how, I asked myself, could I spend money on "silliness" like counseling? Damn! It was all I could do to keep working!

Besides, just like I suggested to the doctor: I was probably: "…just one of those people who are naturally sad."

I had learned to accept it.

To me, people who claimed there was joy in life were just kidding themselves, unable to accept the fact that the world is a dangerous, unfair, unforgiving and dog-eat-dog existence.

Just hours after the appointment, Dorothy and I stood in the dull winter light of our kitchen, where I acknowledged without shame that something was wrong. She had suspected it for years, but we could never imagine how deep it would go, or what would happen next.

Two weeks later, as the doctor promised, I met with a VA counselor. After a one hour discussion she said that it was her opinion that I was suffering from PTSD — Posttraumatic Stress Disorder.

I didn't know what to think. I had heard of some sort of affliction with a similar acronym, yet beyond its curious implication I had no real knowledge of its effects.

The young counselor made an appointment that very day with the clinic psychiatrist for a formal evaluation. Just like her, he said that as far as he was concerned I had PTSD and he recommended I begin treatment.

Treatment?

So I'm having nightmares and feel like crap most of the time!

So what?

Okay — I've had a heart attack and a laundry-list of gastrointestinal issues, mostly attributed I believed to a family affliction of anxiety among our men.

But a mental health issue? A mental *illness* for God's sake!

Man — I don't know. Messing with people's heads? Can't that make things worse? I know a guy who started therapy and they say he ended up in a psych-ward!

But a mental illness? Damn, I don't know.

Could it be possible? Could the nightmares have something to do with this PTS thing?

That evening I read and reread the literature the counselor gave me, underlining areas that I thought might pertain to me.

I was fascinated how my life since Vietnam was exactly like the examples in the brochure.

“This ***is*** me,” I said to myself as I read the VA’s criteria for the disorder:

*__MODULE 1: Re-experiencing__: Intrusive thoughts; flashbacks; nightmares; feeling as if the event is actually occurring — and more.

*__MODULE 2__: **Arousal**: panic attacks; acting out; dangerous behavior —and more.

*__MODULE 3__: **Avoidance**: amnesia; minimizing my experience with others; drug use; numbing — and more.

Not to mention an array of coinciding issues like: survivor guilt; anger; depression; blame; obsessive rituals.

Oh my God!

And on it went:

Problems at work; alienation; distrust of authority; road rage; damaged relationships with family and friends; feelings of worthlessness; feelings of being a failure;

belief in a foreshortened future; intrusive thoughts and flashbacks.

Flashbacks?

Intrusive thoughts?

Could that mean like the thoughts I've had every day where I see myself carrying "him" in my arms? —The dead dismembered young Marine.

I thought that's what went with the territory — You know — going to war. After all, my Uncle Ben was a POW in WWII; my Uncle Joe landed at Utah Beach on D-Day, and his brother John was at Saipan.

And they were OK.

Or were they?

Come to think of it — Uncle Ben drank himself to death.

Come to think of it — Uncle Joe worked himself to death.

And what about Uncle Joe's brother, John? He was in the Marines. When he came back from Saipan he roamed America for two years like a hobo. When he returned home John stayed with us in the country when I was a baby?

Remember mom's stories of how John would patrol the property at night and prowl around the barn with a butcher knife — looking for Japanese?

There was never a doubt that John wasn't "right in the head." But no one ever talked about it.

As I read further, even more familiar symptoms emerged: Things the literature called "Triggers" — like the smell of diesel fuel; burning wood and raw meat; Tastes and sensations, like you have a sixth-sense for danger; even mind-reading of someone's bad intentions.

And lastly: the lack of self esteem; fear of germs; suicidal and homicidal fantasies; paranoia; conspiracies; hyper-vigilance; safety; lack of power and control; loss of trust for anyone or anything — especially of authority or the government.

****

I met again with the VA outpatient psychiatrist in December, 2004. After a one hour discussion he gave me his conclusion in a nonchalant sort-of-way like he had done it a thousand times:

"It's my opinion you have atypical (abnormal) Posttraumatic Stress Disorder and Major Depression," he said.

Holy crap!

The psychiatrist entered the notes of our meeting in his computer and wrote an order for an anti-depressant. He explained as best as he could how antidepressants, SSRI's work, and how in about two weeks I should be "feeling better."

He also recommended that I join a therapy group and I could work that out with my counselor, my 1-on-1.

Only three weeks had passed since I started taking the antidepressants and I was feeling amazingly better. To me, that alone was a miracle and it didn't take long before my family began to notice the difference too, though they avoided, and rightfully so, making a big deal about it to me.

The prospect of group therapy in itself didn't bother me. I knew I could quit anytime I wanted, but I had real misgivings concerning who my fellow group members would be.

Since the 1970's I had seen documentaries and heard rumors of the so-called Rap groups veterans had formed. But these over-hyped and obviously slanted gatherings were the exact thing that made me and many other vets indifferent and suspicious. Not to mention, and I admit, that the last thing I wanted to be involved with for an hour in a closed room were: "…a bunch of loudmouths bragging about how they won the war [my words]."

I was curious though about what it would be like meeting with men with the same experiences. I had spent so many years without male interaction beyond work, it was hard to imagine. But I figured it was worth a try.

I attended my first group session on January 4, 2005. From that first group meeting I was determined to start a journal. I had little expectation of the chronicle other than a lasting record of what could be a special period in my life.

But as the record evolved, the journals took on a life of their own. With each passing year the stack of legal pads increased until they numbered thirteen.

By the time I reached journal number five, in March, 2006, I was beginning to gain a sense of the corrupt thinking which dominated my behavior since that day at the bridge. As I moved forward intellectually, I also opened my mind to the challenges I would face on my path to recovery.

But what is recovery?

Where do we find it? What does it look like?

Will we awake one morning and the trauma and the memories will be gone? Will we prance in circles like Ebenezer Scrooge on Christmas morning?

Surely, not!

Surely, being well and healing and returning to life as a different better person, is something only counselors and psychiatrists believe in.

But not us — We were too far gone!

A month later, in April, 2006, 16 months into therapy, our group was fully involved in a twelve week Cognitive Behavioral Therapy program (CBT). The fifth week of the program an incident occurred just minutes after the session. The lesson this day had mentioned in a small phrase, not particularly relevant to the topic, but it contained a powerful message that moved me:

A "point of wellness," the entry exclaimed. Huh — Interesting.

Accepting and integrating the idea of a concept characterized as a "point of wellness" was something altogether different — It was something reasonable — Something remarkably concrete and successful to pin one's hopes on.

An emotional doorway had opened for me that morning following an incident where I put the lessons of CBT into practice by defusing a confrontation in a manner inconceivable to me previously.

I was struck with the realization that I had achieved, by my definition, a "point of wellness," admittedly one of many spokes on the wheel of recovery, but wellness; a goal; a success nonetheless.

In the journals, points of mending and wellness emerged.

I hope you find yours.

*The journal entries in Chapter VI were condensed for clarity from 13 hand written journals and to focus on the themes.

VI

JOURNALS

January 4, 2005

FIRST TUESDAY GROUP

There were about seven of us. One veteran complained for 5 minutes about not being notified of last week's closing due to weather. Another vet spoke for a good half hour about his ordeal in Nam. He had a large photo of his unit. My counselor seems to look forward to our first 1-on-1 together.

Jan 11

Group discussion on anger. I was very upset. Angry over family issue. Seems counselor believes my reaction comes from stepfather hurting mother. A couple others opened up about their own anger issues. Good session. Feeling bad tonight over taking so much anger into group. I hate guilt. Want to call counselor and apologize.

Jan 12

I was dropping off paperwork at CBOC (Community Based Outpatient Clinic) and saw my 1-on-1 and apologized for outrage. She said glad I did and that's what Group is for. She said another member opened up because of what I said which helped him. That was good—I felt good rest of day.

Jan 18 Tue.

TUESDAY GROUP *Wrote to National Personnel Records Center for my records. In group we continued on anger and how it results in guilt and depression. One member spoke for evidently first time. One other angry and reclused; He feels life has treated him unfairly; Reason why he never had a good job; Says best friend is his dog. He says he has never gotten over girlfriend writing him Dear John while in hospital in Nam when wounded. One guy from New York spent 6 months locked up, as he put it, in a VA hospital somewhere. I told story of day I joined Marines.*

Jan 25

One of the group members spent 15 minutes talking about inappropriate cheek kiss with one of the counselors in group. I left note with psychiatrist K. at reception over his inaccuracies in the notes I recently requested. He said in them: "Mr. McGarrity is doing fine in his work and social life. "WHAT! WHAT WORK AND SOCIAL LIFE? I haven't worked in six months and don't have a single male friend except for my cousin. But I politely pointed out what I thought were mistakes and asked if he would amend them.

*Veterans can request the notes logged at appointments through their local VA facility Release of Information desk.

Jan 27

Called service officer (VSO) and as usual got his voice mail. I said I had my claim package put together and would like appt.

*Shortly after being diagnosed I was encouraged to file a claim with the VA for compensation due to PTSD caused by a service-connected event. By this date I had met with a VSO and he gave me a claim package with a lengthy questionnaire with instructions to contact him when it was completed. Having completed the paperwork in short time which included the dreaded "stressor letter" I attempted to get an appointment with him to go over it.

Jan 31

Still no word from VSO. Called and asked receptionist (whatever, some smartass) if I could have the VSO's direct number. She gave it to me and said in future to call it. DAMN! That makes me mad! Why does it take 5 days to hear nothing then this woman who snickered at me when I came in unannounced gives me a smart- aleck response again. So I left another message for him for an appt. Still mad over his lack of attention I call another County Veterans Service Commission at 2 PM. Told a nice lady my concerns and could I possibly speak to a rep. By 2:15 THE FREAKIN' DIRECTOR called me. He told me I can go anywhere I want to file and he'd gladly see me if I wanted to. Wow! What a relief. So knowing that I thought I'd give another nearby VSO another chance and after Group I'll drop by and make an appt. personally.

*A VSO is a Veteran's Service Officer employed by a county veterans' service office. Along with assisting veterans with filing for benefits they assist in applying for compensation for disabilities. For the most part they are dedicated employees and most often are veterans themselves. They have special access to VA regional offices and receive regular training and upgrading of benefits. In larger cities they are admittedly overwhelmed by the numbers of veterans seeking services.

Feb 11

Appt. with VSO. *He said my claim package was "phenomenal." He was visibly moved by my stressor statement. Said my package will go to Cleveland for adjudication, whatever that is. He says I'll get a letter in about 30 days with a decision.*

* A stressor letter is a personal narrative written by the veteran, which describes in as much detail as possible, including dates, names, units, locations and the circumstances in which he/she recalls the traumatic incident/s or sexual assault/harassment (MST [Military Sexual Trauma]) took place. The stressor is an aspect of the claim process dreaded by many veterans as its contents are

subject to fact-checking by professional researchers at Regional VA claims' centers and the actual writing of the stressor can cause distressing emotional effects during its writing. Some VSO's have questionnaires which help the veteran approach the process at a comfortable pace. A VSO might also recommend having someone the veteran trusts assist them in the composition.

*Realizing the complex issues of having a person recall their traumas in detail, even when the memories are intact, has lead to an exclusion of the stressor letter in some claims' processes.

Feb. 15
TUESDAY GROUP
Counselor asked if anyone had anything going- on that bothered them during the week. I spoke about a local kid I saw in newspaper who had been chewed up in a machine and he lived, but he's gone from waist down. It reminded me of my event in Nam. Another said it reminded him too. One of guys started talking about his chopper pilot experience. He's the only officer in our Group. I felt uneasy, asked if we could slow down a moment. NO! I've done it again. No more. Maybe I should talk about "old Sarge."
Have to speak up. Can't spare others.
*Given the unusual and highly charged politics of the Vietnam War or just a natural inclination for enlisted personnel to dislike and distrust officers or authority figures in general,

it is uncommon to find a mix of officers and enlisted veterans in therapy groups.

Feb 28 *1-ON-1*

Counselor asks how I'm doing? She asked about my relationships with my family? Toward end of group I told her about incident where old Sarge got killed.

*See Chapter II.

March 8

TUESDAY GROUP

Watched relaxation tape for half hour. Not many in the group participated.

*Relaxation tapes seemed boring and unproductive, even corny, taking up important time to discuss issues we faced during the week and were anxious to discuss since we last met. Later I did discover a relaxation technique that seemed to work really well and I still use it to fall asleep.

March 16, 2005

APPT. WITH Dr. K

Mentioned to Dr. K. about his mistake on my notes. He said it wouldn't matter. I told him of issues and stress I was having at my part-time job. That the woman in charge makes me nuts. He noted it.

In the end, the notes the psychiatrist logged about me doing well in my work did become an issue during examination of my claim. Fortunately, I kept meticulous records and this daily journal to counter any misinformation.

Sure enough, the "...is doing well in his [my] work [thing]" came up on my first claim decision. I followed with a NOD, a Notice of Disagreement, which allowed me to contest the finding and I supplied an appointment card and handout material I received from a seminar I attended with Goodwill Industries to use their job-search resources at exactly the same period it was stated that I was "doing well" in my work. This was powerful evidence that helped cancel out the doctor's inaccurate information.

March 29

TUESDAY GROUP

Issues of my event taking on new distressing emotional levels. I'm having dreams where I try to tell wife or counselor about it but can't. I well-up inside as if the words are air rising inside me but can't come out. I learn that though many don't talk in Group, they do talk in their 1-on-1 sessions.

*I questioned my One-on-One on why during group some of the guys never talk.

April 7

Received letter from VA stating they are reviewing my claim and have requested more info.

April 8

Called my local VSO for his advice on the request for more info. As usual I had to leave a voice mail.

April 12

TUESDAY GROUP

Heavy session. Anger—hatred—self hatred. One guy said he locked himself in his room for four days—didn't eat—didn't take diabetes meds. Counselor alarmed. Asked in an irritated way if he was committing suicide. He said wife and him talked about Nam for first time. He seemed happy with that. I got a questionnaire from VA which seems a good sign. I must approach it with absolute clarity—hold nothing back---don't let the fear or images stop me.

April 14

Upset over VSO not getting back to me after week and a half. Two voice mails and a fax.

April *15*

TUESDAY GROUP

Good session. One guy and I talked about him quitting his job. He feels taken advantage of— maybe goes to core beliefs of fairness etc. I told counselor I confronted woman I work for and had told that if she was a guy we would have a problem. I think she recognized it would have taken very little for me to explode.

April 15, 2005

1-ON-1

*Counselor points to my problems with authority, anger, distrust — of what might have caused it. Told her of anger and letdown I felt by officer in the field. Counselor says she feels I have always hated him [*the officer*] and that it comes from my core beliefs being trampled on, about how authority in my mind must always do the right thing yet the "good country kid" in me conflicts with my need to believe the world is a fair place and do what you're told and everything will be fine---but it doesn't. Very interesting.*

April 19

HAVEN'T BEEN FEELING GOOD

CHEST PAINS. WENT TO CARDIOLOGIST. He put me on Isosorbide, a slow acting nitrate. Went to work----all screwed up---confused----light headed. Brief flashes of depression ---anger---shaky---barely slept---absolutely did not remember taking shower this morning --- a blank.

April 29

Returned questionnaire VA sent.
Called VSO --- got voice mail as usual --- left message as usual. Stress building---this will be my last call to him!

May 3, 2005

TUESDAY GROUP

Watch one hour epilogue of vets with PTSD in Hawaii. One very similar story as mine, with explosion and guilt. I'm exhausted.

May ***7, 2005***

HOLY MACKEREL!! HEART ATTACK!!

Crap, **,** *I had a full blown heart attack at 9AM! What can I say---what did it? Stress? — clogged arteries? Paramedics took me to hospital. Dorothy was by my side in ER when I passed out---they took her away and zapped me 7 times. People have asked what it was like—you know—the coming through the light thing. I remember seeming to know that this was it---I was dying, then something in me said: "Not today Marine — fight! I remember taking giant gulps of air---oh My God, like the kid did at the explosion that day ---- then I was breathing deeper and deeper and the light came back, or I came thru it, and I heard the commotion around me and I was alive. I had burns on my chest and back from the paddles and nurses asked: "Are you the guy?" and asked if they could see them. Then I went to another hospital where angioplasties were done.*

May 17

TUESDAY GROUP

The 17th *is significant for me---it's the date I entered the Corps. Counselor tells us about a program that would have us mentor new guys coming in. I think I'd really like to do that.*

May 30

MEMORIAL DAY

I guess this might be considered one of the things they call an anniversary, so a lot of thoughts are running through me. The truth, or at least what I perceive as the truth, is that I always felt as if what I did in Vietnam, that is, being a radioman with a motor company was somehow less of what I felt a real Marine should be. In my mind, because I saw plenty of them, a real Marine was out there in the bush, killing VC [Viet Cong], being dropped off in remote locations, lining up on the trail to head into the bush with full packs, socks full of c-rations, weapons, ammo, knives and grease-paint on their faces. So I did everything I could to come as close to being them as I could. I was the guy who obsessed over being the best radioman in the battalion; the guy who was itching to shoot someone, even though when I was caught off- guard on a listening post in the dead of night as several figures passed by me on all sides in the rain and darkness, I buried my face as deep as I could into the soaked grass and prayed that the CP didn't try to contact me which would give me away and I probably would have been shot or captured.

The Iraq war actually made me feel honorable for the first time about my job in Vietnam as I watched them every day, out on the roads getting the crap blown out of them just like I did.

Sometimes, vehicles in front of me would flip end-over-end from a road mine. Sometimes, vehicles coming at me would blow-up and ones behind me would blow up. On one occasion I volunteered to reach the rear of our convoy by driving a Jeep past a full column of vehicles that were on fire; exploding; some with loads of artillery rounds that would rocket across the rice paddies milliseconds before I whizzed by. We were out there every other day, in the heat, the cold, the rain; thirsty and hungry, just waiting to get the crap blown out of us.

We knew it was going to happen; I just hoped it wouldn't be me or if it was, that it'd be fast. Back at the base at the end of the day we never talked about it. What was there to say?

May *31*
TUESDAY GROUP
Video again of Group in Hawaii. WWII vet in video talked about German Medic he shot and how every morning he sees him standing at the foot of his bed.

June 7, 2005
TUESDAY GROUP
Watched video about an Air Force loadmaster who was alone in the plane's compartment with a load of dead American soldiers en-route to Germany. When the plane started experiencing trouble he freaked. I began telling of my experience in radio and code school and how hard it was, especially when they kept drumming-it into us that we have to save lives. Sometimes at night you could hear the dit-dit-daw cadence of guys mumbling code in their sleep. All I could think of was how in the world can I learn this stuff good enough to save lives.

June 12
Going into hospital tomorrow to have the other artery opened and a stent put in.

June 17
Cardio visit. Discussed short term memory issues I seem to have with doctor's practitioner. She said not unusual given the number of times I was shocked. Found out self

payments for health insurance thru my union going from $500 a month to $640. It just keeps getting worse. I'm scrambling to find a plan just for Dorothy and I'll take my chances with just VA care.
Having difficulty sleeping. Having dreams that I try to whisper what happened in Nam to wife but unable to. ANGER! Every time I see those idiot politicians on TV talking about Iraq. Sadness after seeing so many incidents of bombings. Woke up remembering name out of nowhere of Sergeant at Camp LeJeune I hated and came seconds from attacking one morning. Thank God two friends grabbed me. I think of my event in Nam first thing every morning. Concerned for my safety after heart attack and thinking about buying a gun to carry. I will not be a victim!

June 20
Psych visit
I tell Doc of anger issues, about spurts of Depression, of wanting to hurt person I worked with. He says we often fantasize about hurting ourselves or others but the dynamics change when: "YOU HAVE A PLAN TO DO SO."

June 22
Horrible nightmare last night that I went to a friend's barber shop. Someone asked me what happened in Nam. After a sentence or two I broke down, covered eyes, bent into a fetal position. Each time I tried to pry my arm loose from my face it was locked. Through cracks in my fingers I could make them out staring at me. I was so embarrassed.

June 24

Five women Marines were killed in Iraq today. Part of a civil action team. DAMN these politicians. Why don't they take their daughters down and sign 'em up if they're so tough? Hell no---they just run their mouths.

June 28

TUESDAY GROUP

Bush was on TV this morning saying that our troops' sacrifices are important. My butt, that draft-dodging rich kid who watched us regular kids go to war in the Sixties while he and his snooty friends were getting drunk at Martha's Vineyard.

*During the Sixties and Seventies every 18 year old male was required to register for the draft. It was inevitable that you'd be called in for a physical and given a Selective Service classification rating. The highest was 1A. Every day in every major city in the country hundreds of young men reported for their physical for military service. There were ways to get a deferment at first, like in a job necessary to the war effort or a full time college student or married. But as the war escalated and became unpopular (In 1967, 11,000 kids were killed) families with the financial means and political connections found ways around the draft for their sons by going to Canada or getting sympathetic doctors to pad medical conditions or who knows what else. One means of skirting Vietnam was the National Guard which George W. Bush was able to get

into with family connections. As for Dick Cheney, Bush's Vice President, he had five deferments! During the 2004 election season when asked why he went to such lengths to avoid military service, Cheney told a reporter: "I had other things to do."
What infuriated me wasn't that Bush or Cheney or thousands of other privileged kids never served; what really ate me up was that they and the people around them (who also never served) strut around like tough guys who were all for going to war, when they were the first to avoid the military. To me it doesn't really matter what John Kerry (Democratic Presidential candidate 2004) did or didn't do in Vietnam – the fact is – he went!

July 5
TUESDAY GROUP
One member said "we all need to talk" and another thought that the comment was directed at him so he got mad and said" I'll talk when I want to." That was actually the first complete sentence I've heard him use since I joined the Group.

July 12
TUESDAY GROUP
I complained about $258 bill I got for counseling. At session with 1-on-1, counselor said I have authority problems and that I feed off anger like a drug. I think she's right.

*Until my official diagnosis for PTSD I had to pay co-pays for therapy since I still had health insurance through my union.

July 13

Call Service Officer, of course I get his answering machine---he's sooo busy. I leave my number in case he wants to follow up.

July 16

1-ON-1

Counselor suggests that every day I a reenact the event of 38 years ago at the bridge. That every day I react to the world around me as if it were those hours, on that day, when an authority figure let us down, when suddenly a terrible thing happened. She says that my "vision" of danger is so explicit that I see the possibilities of a dangerous situation way beyond how most people see it. That powerful emotions are constantly at work---comparing---judging---weighing all that takes place around me based on that one day: the loss of power; the letdown; the responsibility with NO REWARD! That's right! Where's my medal? Where's my citation? Where did our officer disappear to afterward so no one could tell the story of what Doc and I did? Why didn't we get asked about him? Where did he go?

July 19

TUESDAY GROUP

Not many there today. Counselor says we are coming to meat of group — that being our trauma disclosures. She asked how we felt about it. How did we want to present it? Silence! Finally I spoke up said "I'm ready, let's do it, I'll go first." After all how bad can it be? I've already ran the gamut of emotions. Some of the guys say they don't want to be judged. I think some are afraid of breaking down. I'm not worried about it. I can do it.

July 25
OBSERVATION
Every day the news is the same. Some kid from America gets blown to bits in Iraq. Some days I just shake my head and turn away, remembering more than ever the day it happened to us. Other days I feel the deep sad feeling in my chest. The same feeling I had when I was at my lowest in depression, like a light within me was dimming. Like something really physical was happening inside me and I couldn't stop it. I feel the darkness in my chest. I realize that these feelings have surely contributed to my heart problems. Now it worries me more than ever. As long as I wake every day with the visions of what happened to me---how can my heart heal?

July 26
TUESDAY GROUP
The book we work from says we will go thru several stages: three are Self blame, victimization, denial. It seems like I'm in all of them. I can't figure it out. Everything---everything is to do with that day in NAM they say, and I don't like the thought of that a whole lot anymore!!! THEN, I open the morning paper and the first thing I see is that a bombing killed four G.I's. There's no escaping it!!!

July 28
OBSERVATION
Repetitive thoughts, avoidance, interference, keep checking if things are OK, if they're safe, if coffee pot off, car doors locked, clothes iron off, if something happens it will be my fault.

Aug 3
CALL TO VA BENEFITS LINE
Called VA line to check on claim. Counselor said they are still waiting on my health records---that it takes time because I was in so many places (ship etc.). For the record I was:

1. *Treated for infection in Nam from using newspaper as toilet paper.*
2. *Sought aid for stomach problems while at Camp LeJeune in 1968.*
3. *Sent to a shrink onboard ship for fighting.*
4. *Passed out in Okinawa after giving blood.*
5. *Hospitalized June 8, 1968 in Everett PA after wrecking car trying to get home on a short leave. Had brain concussion and chest trauma.*

Aug 9, 2005
TUESDAY GROUP
Oh my God! This week 21 Marines were killed in Iraq! Seven Marine Reserve snipers from 3/25 Weapons Company in Brookpark, Ohio were killed. Then 14 Marines were burned to death when a "shaped" IED (Improvised Explosive Device) blew up their 16 ton Amtrac. A big deal was made of their sacrifices with flags, ceremonies, bands, speakers. But in the end

someone's son or husband got the crap blown out of him for a trumped-up war they see as heroic as long as SOMEONE ELSE'S KID! is going to fight for them!
The Tuesday Group is about to reach Chapter 20 where we tell our stories. I'm anxious to prove I can do it. I can see the scene so clearly: the grass, the weather, the smoke, the smell.
My wife Dorothy got a call today from VA inviting her to attend a meeting tomorrow night at the CBOC (Community Based Outpatient Clinic.) I'm proud of her for agreeing to go but it's exactly what I would expect of her. It will really be interesting to hear her response.

Aug. 14
I spent the evening drawing very graphic and distressing pictures of my event. Dorothy seemed concerned.

Aug 15, 2005
Had bad dream last night where I am to meet someone for lunch at a remote stretch of highway. In the parking lot is a pickup with two Marines selling items from the bed. I move nearer and see one is a Lance Corporal and the other a Private. The L/Cpl has on Iraq ribbons. The other has none. I can't see what they're selling. The things are in small boxes. The L/Cpl tells me he has served two tours in Iraq and is going back. He's distressed about it. I wake. Anxious, floods of information.

Aug 16
TUESDAY GROUP
So today I told my story in Group. It was pretty intense. It's hard to tell how the others took it. One guy did leave the room—saying he couldn't listen. Counselor commented on my amnesia for part of event. Were there so many dead Marines to load I just shut down? What did I do? How did I respond in the minutes, hours after? Did the Captain survive? Did we walk to Camp Evans? I think I arrived back at base in a Jeep. That means I would have rode with the other radioman but that part's all a blank. An absolute blank.

Aug 19
1-ON-1
Counselor and I discussed the lost information (psychogenic amnesia). Why didn't we talk back at base? Why didn't anyone question us? Did officer disappear? Did he die? Did Doc and I lead the convoy on to Camp Evans? Did the officer ask to be taken somewhere or was he medevaced? Was he dead? Was he so ashamed of his lack of ability to take charge that at Evans he took refuge among fellow officers? Is this why there were no commendations for Doc or me? If I had a blast concussion, wasn't I wounded? Where's my Purple Heart? But I think you need medevaced to get one. The only indication something extraordinary happened during that period in my records is that my proficiency marks were very high, the highest I got my whole tour. The result---I thought I processed my trauma. Truth is it's just the beginning.

Aug 20 Sunday

More thoughts on memory loss. What happened? Did someone kill him? When I helped unload a truck full of bodies were they from the blast? They were stacked like cord-wood in the back of the truck. Maybe they were from Hue. There were so many.

Aug 29

What happened to the lost hours? Could officer have been dead not frozen? Did someone shoot him? What did I do to the old man with the teapot?

Aug *31*

AKRON GENERAL HOSPITAL

After Group yesterday my blood pressure was sky high and I had chest pains. Nurse at CBOC did an EKG, they called 911 and transported me. Had heart catheterization---nothing abnormal seen ----all OK.

Sept 1 *Constant agonizing over the amnesia aspect of my event must be taking its toll on me. I think I'll take a break from journaling for awhile.*

<u>JOURNAL 3</u>

Sept 7, 2005

I didn't expect to start journaling so soon. I'm exhausted from the constant thinking and analyzing and trying to figure out on my own as I'm doing right now.
I believe: What happened has influenced my entire social, emotional and economic life.

I believe: That I crossed-over mentally at some point in Morse Code school to truly believe what they ground into us, that a hundred lives will depend on us---me.
I remember: My only thoughts and emotions that day were: It's up to me to save them; I passed the ultimate test when others were falling apart.
I know: I have never felt anger for the officer after the blast —I pitied him.
I'm sure: That if I had stepped off the road we'd all be dead.
I always thought: That I should have mentioned the possibility of rockets or explosives we found a week or so earlier.
I believe: I can still feel him in my arms

Sept *9*
EXHAUSTED *Am I here; Am I there; Am I this; Am I that? The depression is better due to drugs but I'm having nightmares. I think of my event every day.*

Sept 23
SUNDAY
Cold morning. Needed to get outside where it's peaceful. I built a fire in back yard and sitting there I had a vivid recollection of a chopper landing at my event and I imagine myself kneeling on one knee into the compartment. That's the first "new" information I've had about what I might have done, other than what I've always remembered. I could feel myself on the deck of the interior and the blades spinning slowly above me.
It brings up a point: Did I lose consciousness at the chopper and got loaded on? That could explain why I

had no recollection of arriving at Evans. NO—the wounded would have been taken one base further north where a full med station was.

Oct 2

TUESDAY GROUP

Another guy processed trauma. Was electrician in Navy. He lived aboard a barge. His job was going around to villages to install generators. One evening he and friends walking back to barge through city with him slightly ahead of others. As he rounded corner a figure darted from a doorway, looked at him and lowered what he said looked lie an automatic weapon. He backed into the darkness and froze as the figure leaped over a short wall and probably ran down a trail into the jungle. When friends arrived he was still frozen. Has terrible guilt that he didn't react.

Another vet in Group was a light artilleryman with 26th Marines at Khe Sanh during the siege of '68. He told how he and fellow crewmen went down into bunker minutes before their gun emplacement took a direct hit from NVA artillery which destroyed the gun and killed the entire crew next to them. For weeks, Khe Sanh was hit with up to 1000 rounds a day.

I have written letter to MOPH (Military Order of Purple Heart) to state my case for same due to blast concussion. At this time it is not considered a wound.

Oct 11

TUESDAY GROUP

Another vet processed his trauma. He was a combat engineer. He hasn't spoken since I joined the Group. He was in an explosion much like mine on his very first day in Nam. He pleaded with officers at base to turn off lights at night near a makeshift volleyball court after repeated rocket attacks. They wouldn't so he decided to take his safety into his own hands and spent the next months sleeping in a bunker away from the rest of his platoon. Veteran (A) who has appeared very upset in the last two sessions has been hospitalized after he requested same from counselor. He says he feels safe in a hospital setting.

*In some entries veterans are identified with a letter like A,B,or C. I felt it was good to use a code for them to honor confidentiality.

Oct 18

TUESDAY GROUP

More trauma processing. Just when you think you heard it all and the Vietnam experience was all insanity, b. s. and bravado, more comes to the surface. I'm not judging and I'm learning that regardless of the story the only thing that matters is that THEY believe it. You be the judge. Vet says he went to artillery training in the Army and after arriving in Nam his first day to his outfit he fell thru the belly hatch of the chopper where a hook caught him and he dangled under it till they landed. When they reached the firebase he was made a cook AND did artillery duty. During an assault by VC he said as he shot his first enemy the VC cussed him out as he died. Then he said that an officer tried to console him and invited him in and gave him a bottle of whisky with orders to drink it all and he did. Then he told of a night when in a foxhole with a buddy he woke in the morning and his friend's head was cut off. The VA currently says PTSD is a traumatic event beyond the realm of normal human experience.

*Memories of trauma can be distorted and fragmented. PTSD complicates them further. What's important I think is that the victim believes the memory.

Oct 24

CALLED WARM LINE

My stressor has been "conceded" meaning it is found "accurate and true" by a fact checker. Warm line adviser says 2 things will happen: It will go to the rating board or I will get contacted to report for an exam by a shrink. This is great news!!!! Thank you!!!!! Thank you family!!! Thank you God!!!!

*Not having received a commendation or Purple Heart for the event, as well as no officer's daily report since he was incognito caused me to describe in remarkable details the location, weather, what names I could remember and on and on. It was a daunting task but in the end a fact-checker evidently uncovered the details of the incident and my recollections matched.

Oct 25

TUESDAY GROUP

(A) is back. He got out of hospital on a Tuesday. Bothered supposedly by some issue with a worthless family member whose story we have heard time and time again. He said he would break his silence and tell his story next week.

Nov1

TUESDAY GROUP

(A) is supposed to speak about his trauma today but wouldn't you know he has a doctor's appt. in 20 minutes. [I was angered]. *"You know (A) my entire schedule revolves around Group. One morning I was sick as heck and made it and another day I limped-in with a screwed-up transmission. BUT I MADE IT TO GROUP!!!"*

Nov 4

AMAZING ENCOUNTER

Amazing encounter this week with two guys from my battalion in Nam. First was a truck driver from 3d Motors I found on internet who left America and is living in Philippines. He remembers driving truckload of bodies to our compound but says it was in February of 68 so that would have been from Tet Offensive in Hue, not my event in Oct. Second was guy who saw something on internet and contacted me. He was a radioman too in my unit and remembers others talking about my event. Later that day he emailed me and said he thinks guy was (John C.) I remember him well, he was a really new guy. That would make sense, being a new guy and all he would have let me and Doc handle it.

Nov 8

TUESDAY GROUP

Group member I will call (A) finally spoke today. He told of how in Nam he befriended a little Vietnamese boy whose village was near where they were clearing terrain. They spent a lot of time together. (A) said he would give him food and send his mother cigarettes. At some point

the boy's mom was killed. (A) said he thought of taking the boy back to America but soon after (A) was wounded. When he returned from the hospital he learned that the boy had been killed. He blames himself for not being able to protect him.
Counselor announces that workloads demand that Groups be merged. I've met some of the people from the other Group and they seem like a bunch of Bush lovers. Not the kind of people I want to be in a closed room with and I tell same to Counselor. Most in my Group think like me that government is full of conspiracies.

Nov 15
TUESDAY GROUP
Counselor opened by exploring our processing over the past couple sessions. But I've been thinking about the whole, not-talking-with-each-other after an ambush thing. Did we really have to? After all, these guys were my family. My real family. They were Mom's kitchen, a soft bed, homemade fudge; the smell of perfume and hairspray. As long as they were there each night, nothing needed said. Maybe the mess cooks would have remembered to light the heaters over the outdoor showers or maybe two or three of us would pull our beat-up lawn chairs into a circle and drink whatever someone managed to get from Mama San with anything we could find, mostly Kool-Aid. We'd sit and drink and chain smoke and laugh till our cheeks hurt and talk about buying a new Camaro or GTO or Dodge Charger when we got back to "the world." We imagined going back to the old neighborhood where high school friends would pat us on the back and buy us beers and promise to put in

a good word in to the supervisor down at the plant. And then, less than a day off the line at Quang Tri, I'm standing in the blazing sun on Okinawa---hours away from going home, and this enlisted guy in charge says that someone named Martin Luther King just got shot and there are riots all over the country. I didn't even know who this Martin guy was. And then he tells you and 100 other Marines standing in a circle in our underwear around a pyramid of discarded jungle fatigues and worn out boots that: "...here's what you'll have to do if you want to carry a weapon (handgun) home with you for your own protection."

WHAT?

A WEAPON?

And he went on: "...go to the PX and pick out the pistol you want then have a chit sent to the Provost Marshall's Office. On your flight, the weapon and ammo must be kept in separate pockets, blah,blah,blah, you'll have to stay here on Okie (Okinawa) an extra day for approval." That was the clincher---an extra day after waiting13 months didn't seem worth it. Besides, it couldn't really be that bad at home— could it? Come on---Hippies beating up servicemen in the airport bathrooms? Old ladies walking up to guys and shooting them in broad daylight? Cities on fire?

It can't be that bad!

So me and a tall Puerto Rican kid and one other guy decided that once we reached San Francisco we'd stick together and defend each other to the death if we had to.

We checked in at the military base at Treasure Island and were taken by bus to San Francisco Airport. We were so hyped-up over the whole riots-thing that as we passed through a tight section of road in the mountains, wouldn't you know, there was a brake-fire and seeing the red glow against the cliff wall and the smoke, I'm sure everyone's thoughts were the same as mine, that: "MY God, somebody dropped an explosive device off the ledge onto the bus."
The three of us walked into the airport about 3 in the morning. The hallways were lined with young people sleeping in the aisles: dirty, unshaven: in the clothes we had only heard about: sandals, bellbottoms. It was like we were on another planet. As promised, we stayed with each other, watching each other's backs until each of us were on our own flight.

I WAS ACTUALLY GOING HOME!

People have asked me what kept us going. I think it was helping the guy close to you keep his dream alive. Each time we sat down together at night or on watch---it was one more day down---one day "shorter"--- one day closer to sweet-smelling girls ----cheeseburgers —fast cars --- pats on the back and a good job and maybe our own apartment.
Then when someone went home we thought of him, and we'd wonder if his dreams had come true.

Then another left and another — each one having a dream that we felt part of --- encouraged-by.
"Hey Ralph, tell me again about that place in your town."
It was hope. Hope for them, hope for me: one day closer. And when they were gone---we promised to write— but we seldom did. We promised to find them when we got back, but if you did, you could feel the tension. It wasn't the same. I wonder if we hated to look the loss of the dreams we shared with them in the eye.
Your dreams were mine---don't ruin them with the realities of not turning out that way. That was our protection---if your dreams became crap, then maybe mine will too — I want you to remember me as the guy who went back to all the things I talked about — and you talked about — and he talked about— even if most of them were lies.

Nov 22
TUESDAY GROUP
I brought up my thoughts on stealing the dream and counselor thought it was interesting but she said those were feelings "outside me." I think that means tell me about what's INSIDE you.

Nov 23
NIGHTMARE
Terrible nightmare! Dorothy and I are in a Jeep and saw the entrance to a large sand quarry was open and we drive in. Suddenly we're surrounded by walls of dirt and sand—the passage grows tighter as we turn a corner where on both sides of us are scattered damaged vehicles

littered on the hoods and beds with the mangled bodies of people in military uniforms with gaping wounds. In a panic I back up and as I swing around we are blocked- in by men dressed in green. A warrant officer approaches and I salute him. It seems he recognizes my characteristic Marine salute and they seem to ease- off the imposing posture. I tell them how we entered purely by coincidence — then I wake up — unable to return to sleep.

* Throughout my years after Vietnam I didn't have nightmares about war. Some find that unusual but it's true. However, I always had violent, very detailed nightmares mostly about being chased by wild animals or that I'm hopelessly lost. Eventually, my wife and I found it necessary to sleep apart as I was thrashing about too much for either of us to sleep well. In 2004 I began experiencing my first nightmares about war with myself as an active participant.

Nov. 29

TUESDAY GROUP

Observation: *Mom remarried and took me from the country. But it didn't hit home until he started smacking her around --- demanding that I work at the golf course. It was the reason I headed for the country as often as I could. The reason I got hit by the car. Oh yeah---250 stitches---shaved head------teeth jammed against roof of mouth; nose flattened like putty---my face the color of ashes. Imagine my first day of high school!!! You wanna talk about core beliefs? Try that day on for core beliefs to* *form: You're ugly; you're no good; the world is a dangerous place; nothing will ever help you recover---- life is hopeless and you are worthless.*

Dec 6
TUESDAY GROUP
Another vet told his story today---he was very agitated. He arrived in Vietnam in 1965. He went over on a ship. He said he was very afraid of the water. He was a wrecker driver. He was once trying to catch up to his convoy, hit a road mine and truck was flipped into a ditch. Night came and no rescue. Could hear villagers mingling around him----was injured too badly to escape-----had to stay in truck all night alone and wounded. He told how he was an alcoholic for 20 years and divorced 4 times. J. seldom leaves his house because he believes his neighbors are plotting against him.

Dec 13
TUESDAY GROUP
Another group member told his story. He started his tour in Vietnam as a stevedore in Danang unloading ships. Then he said he volunteered for something that wasn't quite clear to me and he ended up in a tower on a perimeter somewhere. I shouldn't judge, but I don't understand the stories of guys telling of being transferred out of their MOS's. He says he was put on a small island in the middle of a river with a .50 cal machine gun and ordered to cut any boat in half that violated a notice not to pass a certain point. He says there were quite a few. I guess the truth is, no matter how wild these recollections

might seem it is what they believe! It's not up to me to judge or criticize them.

Dec 27, 2005, 8 PM
I expect this to be my last entry for 2005. It's been a full year now since my first visit to VA. Feeling calm tonight --- like it's gonna be OK.
This might be a good time to look back on where my core beliefs and anger came from. I think my beliefs about fairness and work and authority and responsibility came from my grandparents. I really don't remember sadness as being any part of my life until Mom remarried and the abuse against her started. Tipping point with him was waiting on the porch for him to come home and take me on a much-awaited and planned camping trip right down to the expensive down-filled sleeping bag we ordered from a catalog. "He's not coming Jim," my mom said as I sat on the porch steps watching for him. "Yes he is," I answered. "He promised." After that night it was over with him.

JOURNAL 4

Jan 3, 2006
TUESDAY GROUP
We're exploring spirituality. This seems to be a tough subject. Most of us agree there's a higher power but I said I didn't believe God kept me alive that day. People have always said for what I've gone thru my whole life, God must be saving me for something. If you asked me if I believe in God I'd say yes — mostly because I fear saying no.

Jan 5

1-ON-1

I told my counselor that my new favorite saying is something I read in our book: "Given the person I was and the circumstance I was put- in, I did the best I could." That may not sound like much, but that's a powerful statement for me or any vet with PTSD. Then we talked some about Mom's suicide and how I could apply this lesson and we talked a little about God and my thoughts on being a bad person and about how so many people I've come in contact with have been injured or die.

Jan 8, 2006

Been reading a study Bible my daughter gave me. She suggested starting with John ".....for those with doubts."

Jan 10

TUESDAY GROUP

So somewhere I pulled up this demon of how when I returned from Nam, we were assembled as a mish-mash of Viet Vets and new guys and bunched together for 6 months on a troop ship. It was insane!

Then out of nowhere I started on authority. I guess I was triggered by one of the guys who talked about two things that have bothered me: 1.Not being able to contact Medevacs when we had wounded because I didn't have the right frequency. 2. The incident with the old Master Sergeant --- my feelings of guilt over his death and my fear of being prosecuted. Deep down I was sort of glad they put it on the driver because he jumped out of the truck and that's why we flipped into the water and the

Sergeant died. By then I was rambling — stomping my foot.

Jan 12 Noon

Last night was tough. Tossed until 2 AM. Finally fell asleep around 6AM. Lord please be with me tomorrow.

Jan 13 Friday C&P!

*C&P stands for Compensation and Pension Exam

Wouldn't you know, it's Friday the 13th. Today is a turning point of the past year's journey. Met with a Dr. Z. at 9AM at Mental Health at VA Medical Center. Dorothy waited with me in waiting area and Dr. Z introduced herself and she and I walked to her office. She started by saying: "We are meeting today to examine you for your claim for PTSD." She also asked if I had any problems meeting with an Asian and I said no.

She didn't ask one question like so many veterans say they ask.

She said that we wouldn't be discussing my trauma---that my records have already established that as true and accurate. She said she wanted to know about me as a person. She asked me about my early life. We discussed my happiness as a child until my mother remarried. We discussed her suicide (she asked why she would do that during a divorce) I said she was frightened to death of being penniless without a home. She asked when I first felt being unhappy – I said not long after Mom remarried. We talked briefly about how I felt after the car accident ---I told her I built up defenses to shield myself from hurtful looks and comments. She gradually worked toward my Vietnam experience. I showed her drawings I did of the day at the bridge and she seemed to respond emotionally. She asked me about depression and her most compelling question was: "Do you feel worthless."

I couldn't seem to answer----I searched for the answer. I tried to think that I should say no, but in my mind neither answer made sense—yes-and-no flashed back-and-forth in my mind as I tried to draw one answer in, but I could not. Seconds went by----the words would not come out. I finally shook my head and said: "I don't know."

The session was over in an hour. In closing she asked: "Can you say that what happened to you that day affected your life and always will?" I took a few seconds---looked into her eyes and said: "Based on what I've learned this past year in therapy, I do believe that what happened to me that day in 1967 affected my entire life and always will."
Dr. Z walked back to the waiting area with me where Dorothy was waiting. As we arrived, the Doc said in a soft consoling voice: "You did well." That's an odd statement. Or maybe not, as her job was to establish PTSD and maybe it was her way of saying: You did well proving your claim.
*Awareness and acceptance of having a mental illness are powerful aspects of the "healing" process for those with PTSD.

Jan ***17***
TUESDAY GROUP
What a day! Great news! Requested copy of Dr. Z's comments. OK, news that you have a mental illness

seems at odds with each other, but I'm finally validated. I read report in parking lot. Axis I; Diagnosis: Posttraumatic Stress Disorder Complex and Major Depression partially in remission. Further: "... more likely than not, these disorders were combat-related due to a traumatic situation in the military, causing employment problems and significant hindrance and social isolation.

* For forty years I felt I never deserved to complain. As I have said previously, I was only a radioman in a truck. To have someone who has heard the absolute worst of humankind's afflictions and brutality say that I was affected by a combat related situation, makes me feel something positive about myself.

Jan 24

TUESDAY GROUP

Good turnout. (A) took up most of the session with same problems with his parents. Says he's taking care of them a lot now. We've suggested ways for him to get help but it's like he thrives on his victim status. I told him in a good way that I thought he was setting himself up for failure; that it's inevitable his parents will die then he'll blame himself, perpetuating his victim status. At end of session counselors announce we'll be participating in a special pilot program. I'm excited that what is learned from us helps others.

Jan 30

1-ON-1

Talked a bit about childhood but mostly how I dread November elections ---how these right wing conservative bastards on TV make me feel like someone has my heart in their hand --- squeezing it like a ripe tomato ---the juice---the blood---- dripping out.

Jan 31
TUESDAY GROUP
Good turnout. Pilot program has been postponed till end of February.

Feb 21
TUESDAY GROUP
The Marine who spent night wounded in a flipped truck won't be coming back. Counselor says the heavy meds and agoraphobia (inability to leave the house) has taken a serious toll on him.

JOURNAL 5

March 1
OBSERVATION
Found an entry I wrote about guilt. Here it is more or less. Guilt and blame are the greatest of all pains---that's why I do all I can to avoid it --- perfectionism---hypervigilance. There is no pain greater than blame---regardless if it's a flat tire or a death---they're all the same to me.
Do I blame myself for what happened at the bridge? Sure seems like it. One thing for sure, I blame myself for old Sarge's death.

March 7
TUESDAY GROUP; CPT

(Cognitive Processing Therapy) (Pilot program) begins. First phase of 12 week program. First assignment is writing at least one page called an Impact Statement. One vet is extremely anxious — he wants to back out.

March 14

TUESDAY GROUP; SESSION II CPT

All present. Good job by Member C.

Another vet, J. didn't like having to do it, said he was up till 2 AM struggling with a few sentences. He confides in me afterward that he doesn't know if he can do this. I feel funny about putting so much pressure on the others but that's me. I obsess with details and perfection.

Afterwards we fill out info sheets. I had a lot of trouble with one question: something like: True or False, when things are going badly you are HOPEFUL it will be alright. HOPEFUL? I could not answer it. I asked counselor to help me figure it out. What does hopeful mean in this context?

I read it over and over. The words melt in my mind, swirling, jumbled. For a second I think I know the answer but can't fix it in my thinking or bring the pen down to mark it. I become really frustrated---confused ---- ashamed. WOW! Something really is wrong with me! Then counselor explains it to me in a simpler way, posed the question with less choices. I finally forced myself to mark F for FALSE. That was one of the strangest experiences I've ever had.

* I began referring to terms like *hopeful* and *well* and anything similar as "positive" words which somehow seemed in conflict with my thinking for so long that they were foreign;

almost toxic. It was like positive words were air inside me that couldn't be released. I knew what the word meant and what I should say but was unable to bring it forth. This has lasted a long time and I sometimes still feel a twinge of hesitation when using "positive" words.

March 21
CONFUSION --- COMPREHENSION PROBLEMS
WHAT IS IT? Having problems understanding CPT.
*Again, something in my negative thinking or disruption of logic due to PTSD made identifying faulty thinking a difficult, if not impossible proposition. Other vets were also stumped by the prospect of identifying "faulty" thinking or: "stinking thinking" as some refer to it.

March 23
REFLECTION
*The **authority thing** and my **trauma** are intertwined? Really?*
A couple weeks before the explosion at the bridge, the convoy commander, a Lieutenant, grabbed my wrist which caused me to lose aim a moment before I shot a civilian I believed was setting an explosive. The officer was shocked and admonished me. Then weeks later, at the same bridge when the massive explosion occurred, the same officer froze or had a blast concussion or maybe he was killed. I never saw him again. I never thought of him. I really didn't care. But I never blamed

him for freezing. In fact I always pitied him. I remember being only glad I was surviving, that I didn't lose it like a lot were. I proved I had what it took. While those around me were falling apart, me and Doc were saving lives. Yeah, the reality that the VC and people from the village wanted to kill us really hit home.

So, if my trauma caused me to have an authority problem---how is it that believing that those in authority MUST ALWAYS do the right thing, not trusting authority? Did my beliefs that authority-figures must and always do the right thing and so they ***deserve*** *trust destroyed that day? So that would be why I'm constantly struggling not only with authority but with trust too?*

April 16

OBSERVATION

Went to Easter dinner at sister-in-law's. OK, didn't feel great---mouth really dry—urinating a lot. Really sore in my joints. Had a dream last night that I was lost in a ghetto neighborhood again. It starts on a hill in a big city. I need to get down to the main street. The streets are brick with narrow alleys. In some places steps lead down to other streets---always down. I ask directions-----evil looking people give me wrong ones. They peek out their windows and thru cracked doors. I go down and down. In some places I have to scale down cliffs. Sometimes paths lead to drop-offs and I have to turn back. I wake up sweating.

April 23

Sunday, my birthday

Finding I'm more apt to say: "It'll be good enough like that," instead of: "...it has to be perfect." I hate being a "worry wart," "sad sack." I'm curious why some in Group are resistant to things that will help them. Shouldn't we want to be better people? It's all so mysterious. Why can't I just accept things? Why does it seem there has to be "Golden Words" --- some statement that will say ---- this is what's wrong with you ----- and this is why. Have we already discovered it?

*We were in a war

*It was getting worse

*More and more were getting killed

*I was in the mine truck

*There was an explosion

*Many Marines were instantly killed or dying

*I helped Doc with the wounded

*I directed the choppers in

*I asked the CO about pouring water on Pappy

* I carried disfigured Marine to side of road and dropped him in grass

*There were piles of arms and legs

*I walked toward the old man --- I had a weapon in my hand---I kicked his belongings

*Everything is blank

*I'm at Camp Evans washing the blood off me

*I talk to classmate from high school

*I'm in Phu Bai ----I don't know how I got there ----don't know how much time has passed. My clothes are covered with dried blood

*The guys in my platoon are looking at me.

**And that's that*
** In another incident I told new driver there was contact ahead --- he panicked, tried to grab the speaker—drove off the dike---he bailed out just before it flipped into the rice paddy*
** Old Master Sergeant in the truck's bed was killed. I was in cab covered with sandbags with water to my chin. They pulled me out.*
** I could see Sarge lying in the road --- dead---a bone sticking out of his arm*

April 25
TUESDAY GROUP, SESSION 8 of CPT
Good session. Maybe most productive we've had. I was sort of glad one guy wasn't there who dominates sessions with same stuff. One Group member has a family cabin in PA, has mentioned several times about 3 of us going. Sounds good but I can't do it. If I did I'd want to drive myself so I could leave if I wanted. I honestly just don't have or especially want full time relationships outside of home.

April 30 Sunday
I really do seem to be obsessing less. I hate being the "anxious" guy. In a strange way I seem to have shed something. I imagine another me----a sad me----standing outside my body looking at me. Today I'm reading the book ***The Emotional Brain*** *by LeDoux. It has amazing facts about the physical changes the brain goes thru when trauma occurs. If I get a chance to be a "peer counselor" I want to learn more about how the brain and memories work.*

May 2

TUESDAY GROUP, CPT Session 9

I'm captivated by ***The Emotional Brain****, especially chapter titled:* ***Where the Wild Things Are.*** *It talks about how memories are formed, retrieved, degenerated and fragmented. This is not Philosophy or conjecture but real scientific facts. Too much to go into here but as Group member talk I can see what I'm learning in the book. (A), Today the guy who is always down over parents being taken advantage of by family member is actually ecstatic even clean shaven. Evidently he found a Power of Attorney and was able to remove his dad from hospital. He had won!!! And we were happy for him.*

But counselors questioned his joy and since CPT teaches other ways of thinking they asked him and us to challenge our thoughts using his experience in the Challenging Beliefs Worksheet. Not one of us could come up with anything. I barely spoke this session. I wonder if being quiet is my way of expressing my weariness with (A)'s situation every week.

May 9

TUESDAY GROUP, CPT Session 10.

Talked about self-esteem. I talked about difficulties after car accident as a teen.

May 23

TUESDAY GROUP, Last CPT Session

The 12 week course is over. One vet was deeply distressed---something about losing a ton of money in a legal situation. Did we accomplish anything? I'd say half the guys barely put an effort into it. But I won't judge them any further. Up until about lesson nine I was lost too ---- couldn't make my thinking do an "about face" which is what CPT asks you to do --- to identify the faulty thinking we've lived with for years and challenge it in an assertive, productive way. I was so frustrated. I did finally reach the point in CPT where challenging the "automatic thoughts" in one major exercise made sense but actually saying the words was almost impossible. I had, and still have to an extent a bizarre inability to make positive comments like: I am hopeful; I look forward to, etc. If I had to describe what I got from the 12 week course I guess I'd say that good people---- people who feel less anger or pain, face life's moment-by-moment situations and difficulties thinking about the consequences, whereas we see on some level that this is the right way to conduct ourselves ---- but something in our thinking puts consequences aside. I mean, it's fine to look at a formula and say: "This is how you should act when someone insults or confronts you" --- but walking away will be the test. For me, walking away would be terribly if not totally impossible. I recently challenged my faulty or automatic thinking in an issue with my adult daughter--- it doesn't sound like much but was a difference in our thoughts on spirituality sort of thing --- and I seemed able to picture it from her perspective. That's pretty significant for me. Now I'm hoping to be in the peer program and maybe help others learn how to do it.

*Cognitive processing or CPT, related also to CBT or Cognitive Behavioral Therapy, in my view and by definition teaches us to recognize that our thinking is what gets us in trouble and it drives our behavior. Identify the thinking and the behavior will follow.

<u>JOURNAL 6</u>

* I was so obsessed by the LeDoux book that I felt if I didn't record the things and where to find them, that people might not believe me or that I might lose or forget them.

Joseph LeDoux ---- neurophysiologist professor, Center for Neural Sciences, New York University
P. 228 ... when fear and anxiety impede normal life then a fear/anxiety disorder exists.
P.229 ...The characteristic features of anxiety disorders are intense anxiety and avoidance of situations that are likely to bring on those feelings.
P. 229...OCD (obsessive compulsive disorder)[tries] to neutralize anxiety.
P.230 ...fear conditioning (how about courage conditioning?)
P.231...pain, loud noises, loss of physical support with other stimuli present causes fear conditioning.
P. 233 Anxiety motivates us to deal with traumatic events in advance of their occurrences. Man afraid of elevators takes stairs.
P. 236...evolutionary changes
P.237...ancestral fear conditioning
P.239...multiple memory systems-----hippocampus and amygdala.
"Trauma learning" is the result of conscious memories by hippocampus and unconscious memories by

amygdala. When trauma related stimuli are encountered---- conscious memories come back through the hippocampus and the amygdala prepares for danger. But the amygdala, the ancient fear-conditioned part of our brains has "learned" to override the hippocampus and its logic when trauma occurs and it "says" NO, this is not a logical situation----this is danger---life or death danger and we must fight or flee or freeze.
P.240..... *hippocampus suffered a stress induced breakdown during trauma due to adrenal overload. When stressful situation occurs the adrenal gland secretes steroid hormones into the blood to mobilize us.*
P.241...*hippocampus is like a thermostat, its receptors receive the stress hormone and tells the hypothalamus to "slow down" the release of the ACTH chemical which activates the adrenal gland to release the stress hormone: adrenaline. This cycling helps balance the demand of adrenaline with the need. However, if stress persists too long, the hippocampus begins to falter in its ability to control the release*
P.242 ...*With prolonged stress, IRREVERSIBLE CHANGES TAKE PLACE. Cells in the hippocampus actually begin to degenerate. When this happens the memory loss is permanent.*
In survivors of trauma, like with PTSD, the hippocampus is shrunken with deficits in memory.
P.244...*If the hippocampus is completely shut down by stress where it had no capacity to form a memory during the event --- then it would be impossible to retrieve a conscious memory of the event.*
P.245 *The only clear thing about memory-recovery in real life is there is no way for outsiders to determine if a*

particular memory is real or fabricated without solid evidence. It doesn't mean it's false----just distorted. Memories of traumatic experiences can become unconscious sources of intense anxiety that potentially exert their opaque and perverse influences THROUGHOUT LIFE!!!
P.257 *Factors combine and bombard the amygdala with electrical and chemical signals; potent reinforcers of Pavlovian fear conditioning. These powerful stimuli link with the sights, sounds, and smell of battles which also reach the amygdala. Later the occurrence of the same conditions (related stimuli of sights, sounds etc) elicit profound fear responses by reactivating the powerful (fight or flight) amygdala circuits. This gives rise to anxiety and worry like a runaway train.*
We are therefore reacting to danger instead of thinking about it.
WOW!!!! That's some heavy stuff!!!!!!!

JOURNAL 7

June 5, 2006
Reflecting on aggression:
I was definitely extremely aggressive after car accident in 1968 just before my battalion went to the Mediterranean to conduct landing operations and train NATO troops. I had a brain concussion diagnosed at the hospital in Everett, PA. But also in first grade in Florida I was hit between the eyes with a full blow from a baseball bat. I had a nightmare that DEATH was behind a curtain waiting for me. At age fifteen I went through a

car's windshield when I was hit from behind riding a bicycle on a busy highway. In Nam I was extremely close in proximity to numerous explosions.
Acting out afterward: fights in almost every port we went to. Punched a Marine in a bar in Izmir, Turkey, knocked-out another in a Mike boat after liberty. Heavy drinking----experimenting with drugs. Friends eventually wouldn't go on liberty with me. Lashed out at NCO (Non commissioned officer) in troop compartment and was barely restrained by friends during an attack on a Sergeant.

June 11, 2006 4:59 AM

I messed up and forgot to order depression meds. It's been 3 days since I took any. Can't believe how I'm already feeling the effects. Can't sleep. Thoughts racing. Nightmares where I see myself in combat but I'm old with white hair sticking out over each ear like Clarabell the Clown. Me and another guy are running up a hill in a town-----dirt road----our compound is just ahead. I'm carrying an antenna. There are many blown- up buildings all along the right side-----there are snipers in them-----we make it to the top. I'm in water, swimming toward shore. There are explosions all around me. I make it to the beach and run thru a field of tall grass like the field where we played when I was a kid. Rockets are landing all around me ---- I run and run and dive to the ground.
I call VA pharmacy and get a former Corpsman who was at Khe Sanh about same time I was. He says he can help me.

* There's a special connection among anyone who was at Khe Sanh near the DMZ as it personified combat and sacrifice in actions against North Vietnamese Army troops.

June 13
TUESDAY GROUP
Meds working. Starting to feel better

June 26
1-ON-1
Talked about victimization. A victim by definition is a person who suffers from a destructive or injurious action. Every trauma-victim loses something; their innocence, a belief that the world is safe; that people can be trusted. To get out of the victim stage you must restore your self esteem. I must restore my self esteem.

June:
Did I stop Mom from being hurt any further?
Did I save some of those guys because I took charge?
It wasn't my fault they bombed us. I never could have known.
Did my actions cause old Sarge to die? — Maybe.
Can I live with that? — Maybe.
Did I kill the old man at the bridge that day?

June 27
TUESDAY GROUP
Group discussed intimacy. Members especially angry over a situation one of our counselors had with a Viet vet at a clinic in another county recently. She told us about

how this guy goes to family functions and a female family member always says there's no such thing as PTSD in front of the whole gathering. He leaves. We all feel that the relative is a jerk who has gotten away with this, and if most any of us were there she'd be pulling a plastic fork out of her neck.

July 10
1-ON-1

Discussed events of Master Sergeant dying when truck went off road into rice paddy. I have always felt guilty. She says: words are only words-----people make choices and the driver jumped out on us. July 21 Meds increase. I show my meds-manager the drawings I did of event. She raises Sertraline from 100 mg. a day to 150.

*By saying that words are only words the counselor was attempting to tell me what I would later learn was that no one can make someone else do something they don't want to do just through words. That just because I said there's a firefight ahead was not enough to make the driver reach for the radio or jump out on me. That people make their own decisions on their actions.

July 27
1-*ON*-1

Trying to remember what happened that day. The truth is she says that I may never know or remember what happened. More important to focus on what I do know. That I should accept that a physical change occurred in my mind; accept that I may never remember; accept that, and this is big: GIVEN THE PERSON I WAS AND THE CIRCUMSTANCES I WAS PUT IN ---- I DID THE BEST THAT I COULD.

August 22
TUESDAY GROUP
Just learned that my claim was sent to Washington for a STAR Review! Literally, my whole file was sent there to be looked at to see how it was examined and if I got a fair evaluation. That means more delay!
*The review came back showing that it had been reviewed properly.

September 12
TUESDAY GROUP
Traumatic Bereavement Worksheet. I find it confusing ---- especially about self esteem. (A) broke down, says he wants to just die and get it over with.
I'm pretty tired of the guessing games with assignment and so are others------ always conjecture----no results---- depression, anger, shame, low self esteem ---but how do they tie in? Tired of guessing. Need to concentrate on facts. Not my job to figure this out.
FACTS:
Born 1947, happiest kid on earth, few friends, don't really need any, by a fluke in geography I attend school with rich kids, I see myself off to the side alone, I daydream in class, travel to Florida with grandparents where I finish first grade. Heading home we were marooned for a night on a sandbar in the Everglades as the tide surrounded us. When we arrived home grandfather dies; I saw grandmother put pennies on his

eyes. Her, my mom and I move to country, I love it, lots of friends and adventures. When my grandmother died mom marries. He owns a business, seems to have a lot of money, I figure we'll continue living in country, but everything changes, we move to apartment in the city, summer comes, he insists I work, I start to caddy, he forgets about fishing trip and I'm left waiting on porch. He starts hurting her; I hear banging at night --- don't know what it is, I don't know how men and women act when living together. Mom is sad, nothing she does pleases him, she asks me to just try and do what he wants. I begin sleeping on porch, wake up early and hide around block till he leaves. I realize I can ride my bike to the country where I meet with old friends. Sometimes I have to call her to bring me home. She's angry but it's worth it to be away from the city. Then we move even further and I can't get to the country anymore.

OBSERVATION

I believe that:

One day in 1967 something happened to my mind when a bomb went off near me. Because of that explosion and the horror of what I had to see I experienced a chemical overload and began to react to the world around me with guilt, anger, aggression, lack of trust for authority, anxiety, hopelessness, failure, perfectionism, distrust of my decisions, intrusive thoughts, nightmares, hatred, horrible depression, fear of responsibility, obsessive behavior.

SINCE GOING TO THE V. A. IN NOVEMBER 2004:

Medications have reduced the depression considerably. Group has given me something to look forward to each week. I take more personal risks. I actually feel like I WANT to live and enjoy life.

<u>JOURNAL 8</u>

October, 2006

Started a weekly therapy session in our Group with a Dr. Mc. Program is called Image Rehearsal Therapy or IRT for dealing with nightmares. She's really great. Something about her voice is comforting, reassuring, yet she stays focused on the work and no b. s. with assignments or participation from group members. Perfect atmosphere for me.

November 9

OBSERVATIONS

Nearly 2 years now since going into the system: Group therapy, 1-on-1 counseling, CPT and now IRT. Recently had quite a revelation. I guess you'd have to experience the images that I have every day. For the most part they never vary one ounce, leaving me always questioning and probing the image for new information but it never comes. I guess mostly I'd like to see who the other radioman was, where the time went and mostly, what happened to the officer after he froze and we started cleaning things up. But this is pretty big, the first time ever anything was realized and that was the position of the vehicles on the road as we stopped. I realized that we would have stopped to the right --- of course. But what makes it significant is that the vision of me walking to the side with "him" in my arms is distorted because of the fact of where we were sitting and how far I carried him. Also, none of the wounded would have been at Camp Evans, our destination, they would have been taken north to Dong Ha where Delta Med had a field hospital in the Marine Compound.

November 17

1-ON-1

Counselor and I discussed "where I thought I was in therapy." I said I felt like I was in some transition point. She said she and other Group facilitator discussed having me sit-in on another Group in February as a "mentor." I think that would be great.

OBSERVATION

In writing this I hope to give words to the thousands who have searched for their own but were unable to find them. That now I am aware and know that from this day forth regardless of how I deal with the world, even with things as mundane as seeking services or eating in a restaurant, certain facts will always be my companions on the razor's edge of life with me: THEY ARE:

**I will always have PTSD, a mental illness.*

**It will forever define who I am but it doesn't have to control me.*

**I expect it will always be necessary to challenge my stuck points.*

**I expect I will always, at some time each day, see myself standing on the edge of the road with him in my arms and feel the twinge of hurt in my chest.*

March 28
MEET WITH PEER TEAM LEADER
The Center for Stress Recovery (CSR) is located at the Brecksville VA Medical Center in Brecksville, Ohio just south of Cleveland. I meet with Team Leader for an interview to begin the Peer Counselor Training. Under the program, veterans with PTSD and coinciding mental health issues will be trained to go back into their communities and volunteer as co-facilitators in local VA Community Based Outpatient Clinics' (CBOC's) mental health settings----most likely in Groups with a professional social worker as the facilitator. Schooling is every Friday for 2 hours. We will also be trained for 3 full days in WRAP (Wellness Recovery Action Plan.)

April 10
TUESDAY GROUP
We spent whole session on same person's family dilemma, the whole nine yards of his self-described miserable existence. Coincidentally he says he has same VSO as me, the one who never returns calls. I tell him he should get another.

April 11, 2007
1-ON-1 and I'M ACCEPTED IN PEER PROGRAM!
I got accepted in the peer program! Start sessions on April 20 and will go for 18 weeks.

April 20
PEER TRNG.
First day of peer training. There are 16 of us. Some have incredible credentials --- for instance: Masters in

Economics, another in business, another computer science. We introduce ourselves. Interesting stories. One a woman Marine, another woman was one of the first women on Navy ships. The men---Oh Man! One Marine with numerous awards also bi-polar. One Air Force disarmed nuclear bombs. One Iraq vet was a squad leader on convoys---has a high profile job but can't shake thoughts of Baghdad and bombings----arrested for driving on median to avoid dead animals because in Baghdad the enemy puts explosives in them.

April 27
PEER TRNG.
Two peer candidates have dropped out. Mostly more orientation and discussion on some of what we might do in our communities. I'm excited about what my two counselors in Akron might have in store for me.

May 4, ***2007***
PEER TRNG.
Dr. T. gave presentation about dynamics of counseling like boundaries, also drug and alcohol issues. A lot of emphasis on "new model" of psychiatric care ----- the provider/consumer relationship where the consumer plays a more active role in the recovery process.

May 8
TUESDAY GROUP
Worked some on Spirituality. One counselor asks if one of us would like to sit in on a fairly new Group and would one of us like to offer our experience to them. Of course I said yes.

May 11

PEER TRNG.

Anxiety disorders----symptomology----therapy concepts. Pretty interesting that the LeDoux concepts were mentioned.

May 29

TUESDAY GROUP

Working on "goals and values." Seems very hard concepts for us to grasp.

RECAP May25

PEER TRNG.

Discussed psychoses: schizophrenia, bi polar disorder (that's a nasty one, I think that's what Mom may have had).

Oh yeah, began doing something I always wanted to do --- I had procedure done on scar that runs across entire forehead to try and reduce its appearance. A dermatologist basically worked an instrument under it and freed the old scar tissue from where it had adhered on the skull. More to come. Still swollen around left eye and slightly numb over eyebrows. Slight headache still. I think next I'd like to see about permanent bump over right eye. A lot of people have noticed the bruising and when I tell them what I did they say: "What scar?" Isn't that ironic? They say they don't see them but I do.

June (?)

PEER TRNG.

Mostly neuroscience stuff by a PhD. Forehead healing nicely ----still some occasional pain.

June 5

Second full day of WRAP training

More into WRAP now. Bipolar Marine continues making what some in the Group consider condescending comments and sexual connotations. One of the women says aloud that he gives her: "...bad vibrations."

June 6

LAST DAY OF WRAP

Got certificate for completing the course. Scar healing. It has really reminded me of when it happened---the sensations are very similar. There does seem to be some correction in its appearance.

June 12

TUESDAY GROUP

Feeling more and more frustrated with original Tuesday Group in Akron, mostly because of (A's) constant, unresolved family issues. I'm not sure what to do. I enjoy seeing the guys and having something to look forward to on Tuesdays but the peer training has put me on another level of thinking from them.

June 14

STRANGE MAN

I stopped by the village hall where I live today and was talking to two women workers I know in the back office. The police clerk had stopped by earlier and mentioned that a frazzled guy, about 60 with a beard and Border Patrol hat was roaming around town handing out fliers and ranting about the local library board. Wouldn't you know, he came in the building and started in on them about it. As he became more agitated I interrupted him and said calmly but assertively, why don't we go down the hall and talk about this and he agreed. By the time an officer appeared from the nearby P.D. I had the man sitting and the situation de-escalated. It was very empowering. WOW! What a sense of confidence and boost to self esteem. I was calm and assertive and what was becoming intense was neutralized. WOW!

June *19*
TUESDAY GROUP
Good group today. Even (A) didn't complain. We talked about triggers after one veteran complained about how a staff member did what he said was a bad job drawing blood. Conversations went many directions ----mostly about our own triggers --- traumas, core values and their affect on those with PTSD.

June 27
1-ON-1
I told Counselor how I feel like a man without a country; floating somewhere between peer vet and Group member and don't think I'm getting anything from Tuesday Group anymore.
She says she and other counselor would like to try me as a peer facilitator in a group where anger and aggressiveness has ruled. I thought it would be perfect.

July 3
TUESDAY GROUP
Learn I will be introduced as the first peer to join a Group in Akron on July 11.

July 6, 2007
PEER TRNG.
Role playing.

JULY 11
MY FIRST PEER SESSION, [PEERED GROUP]
Wow — enlightening and humbling. Six guys in the Group today. I was so pumped I tried to put all my current 10 weeks of peer training into effect and I guess I pretty much blew it! Didn't discuss session beforehand with counselors or recognize that the two counselors have worked together many years and had what some refer to as: "a style." In debriefing one counselor says I looked nervous. I don't think I was at all. Next session I'll try to settle back----let counselors lead.
*I understood that counselors and facilitators usually met before a Group to discuss how the session might unfold and what they would try to touch-on. Afterward, it's typical for counselors to debrief on how it went and if anyone was in particular need of help. I met with the counselors on an occasion or two before groups but that changed. I think that for all the good intentions on both parts, neither they nor I had a clear idea of how I would participate in the Group as a co-facilitator.

July 13

PEER TRNG.

Session as a peer still bothering me so I shared a fact with fellow peers about checking with facilitators prior to being a peer on what their "Style" is, like: Gestaltian or Adlerian. I think in the end it was a valuable experience and critique, and it will make me a better Peer Specialist (that's the name we are now being officially called).

July 17

TUESDAY GROUP

Same old crap. (A) was stuttering today, had trouble organizing speech after Group. Main counselor absent. Nurse mental health counselor offered encouraging words about my first session as a peer and plans to email my Team Leader about it. Her exact words were: "so far so good."

July 18

PEERED GROUP

Spent more time observing how the two facilitators operate. One vet talked about how he could remember where people who died were from (their home state) but not their names. He was perplexed. I took the opportunity to say that there might be things he will never remember---that memories are fragmented and distorted for a reason.

July 24

TUESDAY GROUP

Wasn't really excited about coming today. Expected SOS, Same Old Stuff. Surprise! Counselor introduced Mindfulness Program: "being in the now:" Being an objective observer of your own experience.

July 25

PEERED GROUP

Went well I guess. Feeling somewhat more relaxed. Have to keep in mind that these guys are in new territory and I'm reminded that I should go slow with them. I suggested that Trust was a Stuck Point of trauma and that seemed to confuse them. A concept they evidently aren't ready for.

*According to an aspect of CPT, there a five Stuck Points of trauma: Safety, Trust, Intimacy, Power/Control, Self-esteem.

July 30

TUESDAY GROUP

(A) in Wade Park VA Hospital. He had a heart attack. I knew there was something going on. Guess he's having a bypass.

August 1

PEERED GROUP

WOW! We're really opening new pathways here. I thought session went OK. There was freestyle talk about tennis shoes that guys bought made in Vietnam. Counselors laughed and so did guys. Chapter 3 asks vets to look at themselves for the person they were before the

military; especially the effects of basic training and boot camp. One vet talked of his All-American-boy upbringing; that life was good and fair and rewarded hard work and ethics. Others said their lives very different. I said how about having someone talk whose life sucked growing up and in military. Counselor liked the idea. One guy quick to volunteer ---he was raised by grandparents---no father---said he quit school to join Marines and graduation was the greatest day of his life. Then went into brief comment of explosion in Vietnam and stopped.
I added that we own our life's experiences in a very individual way and its effect on us is ours and no one else's. At end, vet (Y) volunteered to speak next week.

DEBRIEF: *Counselor liked how I suggested a contrasting narrative. Seems I'm really flying by the seat of my pants now. We discuss if when Group begins processing their traumas, if I should too. Question is: Am I a member of the Group? Counselors seem to agree with each other that I am not.*
But what am I? Counselors agree I'm somewhere between being a group member and a staff member but how should the Group see me? Will they trust me if I'm set apart? Will there be a "better than us" factor? Maybe I should give them their time without me before Group. Maybe I shouldn't be in their "circle." If I see them beforehand it's hard not to react to their conversations. Maybe this violates a boundary. Should I inject myself into their sole domain as a Group?

August 3
PEER TRNG.
OK, I ask an instructor at training and he said NO! He says that the peer should not do reflections on childhood or trauma processing in the Peer facilitated Group. Reasons: He said that once the peer discloses faults, weaknesses, hurt, pain, shame, guilt etc, his or her vulnerability is shown --- he becomes someone who is no longer seen as a helper or guide because he is a hurt person too and how can he help?

August 8
PEERED GROUP
Went well. I arrived purposely at the last moment to avoid contact with the Group members beforehand. (Y) talked as promised. He said he grew- up in a good two parent family. Was sort of a street kid, said his mother "pushed" him into the Marines and he said he was glad she did. He said he spent 20 years in the Corps. Another recalled bad life growing up. He wasn't in Nam but was a morgue tech in Korea. He seems to minimize his trauma as undeserving of the same recognition as combat vets. We assured him how much courage it took to tell us. I made sure he knew that no one's trauma is more important than another — that trauma is trauma.
* It's common for veterans who were not in combat, yet were clearly traumatized, to feel they are undeserving to claim PTSD, at least on the same emotional level as their combat counterparts. The truth is, that whether domestic violence or child abuse or sexual assault or torture or natural disasters, traumatized people will display the same symptoms.

August 15
PEERED GROUP
I'm chomping at the bit to tell them why examining their lives before the military is important --- but I can't----- not yet. One member angry over being questioned ---- he says to staff: "...you're the experts, you tell me why I have this. Don't ask me to figure it out."

August 22
PEERED GROUP
In debriefing after group, Counselor was curious about me mentioning that I was depressed for two days especially after I told her that while reading the Anger chapter, I had a powerful yet unidentifiable vision of the unknown radioman. I envisioned him standing in the road --- staring at me----blank ---- I can see the officer sitting in the Jeep ----frozen. But what if I never do figure out who other radioman was? Will it matter?

August 24
PEER TRNG.
We graduate next Friday after 19 weeks. Team Leader will meet with us individually and discuss contacting our community counselors with a peer plan.

August 29
PEERED GROUP
Been in this Group for 4 weeks now as a peer.

September 6
PEERED GROUP
A group member verbalized his thoughts on suicide and disclosed that he planned to steer his car into the path of any oncoming vehicle. Counselors called for a triage nurse and one counselor exited room to speak with him privately. Outcome unknown.
*The veteran did what the counselors caution about: he disclosed a plan to kill himself and others --- not just a fantasy. I understood that before the clinic could allow him to leave he was required to sign a "contract" not to follow through with his plan.

September 12
NEW 1-ON-1
My counselor, who I've had since my first Group in 2005 is transferring. I will be meeting with Dr. Mc

Sept 19
FIRST WITH Dr. Mc
Met with Dr. Mc for first time. We processed what has been occurring lately in Groups. We covered a lot in 30 minutes.

Sept 25
TUESDAY GROUP
Groups are merging. We're supposed to decide what Group we want to join. I'm not sure I even want be involved with Groups anymore.

Sept 28
I have pretty much decided no to continue with Groups.

Oct 3

OBSERVATION

What is pity like the kind I had for officer? According to Nietzsche (philosopher): pity causes an otherwise normal person to feel his or her own suffering in an appropriately intense and alienated way. I pitied the officer---so I felt my own suffering in a way that was improperly intense, against accepted standards ---withdrawing from the objective real world rather than experiencing the thoughts and feeling associated with reality.

And so, I withdrew from the real world to a place where thoughts and feelings don't exist. Here, I could keep going ---- I was heroic----stronger than many around me. Not better----just stronger.

Oct 8

MY LAST TUESDAY GROUP

Oct 19, 6 A.M.

Last night I read in ***Trauma and Recovery*** *how it's vital for a victim to receive support and compensation from his/her community.*

So how would that pertain to me and my experience? Afterward I was sent away----isolated from the unit---why? Was it so my story wouldn't be recorded? Where's my medal?----my commendation? --- my promotion? I was the guy who saved people----who drove past burning vehicles with exploding shells----that officers asked for ----yet I'm still a lousy E-3 sent to an outpost alone and this loudmouth new- guy from Long Island or wherever gets promoted to Sergeant.

Then I get back to the states and non-combatants are telling me what to do. I risked my life so others could succeed? High school friends are about to graduate from college and will have careers while I'm scratching my butt in the unemployment line.

<u>JOURNAL 11</u>

November 9, 2007 Friday

I got a "calling" today to help someone. There's a place called the Hope Café in a tough section of South Akron that helps street people and the downtrodden. It's one of the poorest neighborhoods in the city. I used to hang there a bit as a kid. It was almost noon when I walked in---I talked to a woman who looked like she was in charge and I gave her $10 and told her the Lord or something powerful had told me to stop by. She invited me to their free meal later to meet some of the folks. I wondered if after so many years I still had what it takes to go into a neighborhood like that at night by myself. Later that evening I drove back. It's dark as I approach the exit. I can see the red and blue lights of police cruisers reflecting along the rows of ramshackle brick buildings lining the neighborhood's main drag.

No big deal---it's Friday night in the hood! At the traffic light a half dozen people are mingling outside a deplorable Greyhound Bus depot. Through a large window facing the street I can see a petrified Amish woman (many come to Akron from southern counties when family members are in the hospital) with wide eyes, sitting in a molded plastic chair with what looks like a pillow clutched tightly on her lap. A young woman walks by with a skirt so short you can almost see her butt-cheeks. The Amish woman is paralyzed with fear.

Three blocks down at the Hope Café, an Alcoholics Anonymous-type joint that serves cheap coffee, a line has formed on an open stairway barely clinging to the outside of the converted two-story inner-city house. The people standing in single file on the stairs in the darkness are there for the free Friday meal, which for most of them is the only food they'll get this evening. To keep themselves a bit warmer while sleeping in makeshift camps and doorways, they'll pack down as much sugar as they can —case in point, all that remains of a donated sheet-cake covers a large rectangular paper platter. A man with a plastic trash bag stuffed with all he owns uses a half-loaf of day-old bread to squeegee the last of the frosting from it.

The pastor is in his early 30's with distinctive Creole or Native American features. He sits at the head of a rectangular cafeteria table in a back room and states that this is a ***Celebrate Recovery*** *program, but it appears he just downloaded the basics off the internet. Four of the men at the table were recently released from prison. A woman in her forties fears being alone in her apartment and so she'll hang around till closing time. A black guy claims to be a Marine stranded between V.A. hospitals and claims he's trying to get back to Pennsylvania. He said he was at the Greyhound station and a girl told him about the free meal. He has an ugly scar on his face and says it was from Iraq. There's a lot of fakers out there so*

I gave him a couple questions only a Marine could answer properly, and he passed.

WOW! *This is Masters Degree stuff. The Marine and I talk afterward. He needs to get back to Pennsylvania. Says he needs forty dollars for the bus ticket. I'm torn---is he scamming me? If I give him the money, will I be a sucker?---a chump? Who cares. Tonight I'll do what I feel is right, even if I am a sucker. He thanked me. It's late----my vehicle is not far but it's in a dark gravel lot. As I leave the building I can see cars speeding by on the freeway through the thin corridors of dark alleys. A noisy crowd of street people have gathered in an empty lot nearby. I'm ready for anything as I walk to my vehicle — I have a large knife in my back pocket. I feel a real sense of achievement as I drive home to my safe quiet place in the country. I did it.*

Jan 7, *2008*
***PEER TRNG*.**
We've been asked to write down some ideas that some new vets coming into the system might like to know, like:
**What are the side effects of the meds—especially sexual*
**Will the meds make me feel high/drunk*
**Will I feel the meds "kicking in."*
**Can I go crazy from the meds*
**Will I have to pay for meds*
** Will I be billed for therapy*
**What do I tell my family about this*
**I've often heard veterans say: "You'll get worse before you get better." What does that mean and should I be concerned.*

I can't remember parts or most of my traumatic event. Is that OK? Will someone try to* ***make-me* *remember.*
**What if I freak out*
**Can a psychiatrist commit me/lock me up*
**What will happen if I fantasize about hurting someone or myself.*
**Will I become a different person*
**What do I tell people who say: "Get over it."*
**Will I have to go to detox before I begin therapy*
** Will my family be involved*
**What is recovery*
**What if my employer says I can't have time off work to attend*
**What happens during the diagnosis and what's this computer-test thing that everyone talks about*
** What is a stressor letter*
**Is it true that meds can take depression away*
**What are triggers*
**Some guys in my Group never speak — why is that*
**Why do some people develop PTSD and another person in the same circumstance doesn't*
**What will happen if I stop taking my meds*
**Sometimes in Group I want to scream at this one guy-----what do I do*
**What's a GAF score*
**I take meds but I don't feel any better — why not and what should I do*
**What is a C&P*
** If I'm declared to have a mental illness like PTSD, will I be on a list that can keep me from having a firearm or hunting license*
**I feel mentally exhausted — is that normal*

March 12

Anger issues. I've been explosive the past few weeks. Went berserk on a girl in traffic today. She was talking on phone, caused me to miss an opportunity to pull out of a busy lot. Mad all day about it — chest pains — back pains. I had to lie down for almost 2 hours. I have overlooked appealing to God and so I will.

April 7, 2008

PEER COUNCIL

Have had less and less to say lately. Team Leader at Brecksville's Mental Health Wellness Center seems to understand how anxious I am to start something as a peer, but he also seems to think it's important that he match me with a Group that at the same time, can serve me as a member of the group myself.

***Observations**:*

**I accept that my anger is a result of my "event."*

**I accept that I have authority issues that are related to my "event"*

**I accept the scientific findings that mental illness is a biochemical effect*

**I accept that people with PTSD have varying levels of cognitive impairment*

**I put tremendous yet unrealistic expectations on authority to do the right thing. But few can succeed.*

**I feel that behavior issues that resulted from my PTSD can be managed but not eliminated.*

**I accept fully that those with PTSD have and gravitate back and forth between 5 Stuck Points: Safety, Power and Control, Intimacy, Trust, Self esteem*

**Now that I want to live, I have become aware of mortality; I'm sentimental about my youth; I want to do good things for people.*

April 12

End of Life *Seminar in Cleveland with emphasis on Veterans. Near end, room was darkened and patriotic-type orchestral music accompanied a slide show of veterans from all wars. I broke down---sobbing----some of the group members attending had to leave the room.*

April 14

PEER COUNCIL

For lack of a better name I have named the gathering of about a dozen peers from previous training with those of us from most recent training as the Peer Council. We meet every Monday at the MH Wellness Center to discuss peer issues, report on our latest assignments, make recommendations and help design curriculum etc. for new vets coming-in and for existing groups and programs.

Ran across an article with this info in it:

Iraq War 5th Anniversary
3,991 dead
29,400 wounded
1.031 amputees
$608 billion spent
30% Exhibit PTSD
20% diagnosed with full PTSD
3,659 children parentless; mostly fatherless

May 6

1-ON-1

Dr. Mc has asked me what I might like to work on. I've been thinking a lot about it. I feel I'm straining to attach some kind of distress to my life so we can have a dialogue about it. But each time I do this, Dr. Mc offers words of comfort — sometimes having me see things in a positive way, challenging my thinking with clear lessons like: ".....you can't help how you feel, but you have choices how you act on the feelings."

WHILE I'M LOOKING FOR REASONS TO FEEL BAD — Dr. Mc. OFFERS REASONS TO FEEL BETTER.

June 16, 2008

***FIRST REAL PEER ASSIGNMENT*!**

Due to a new, more efficient system to bring veterans into the Center for treatment, the Center has established a system where referrals by VA doctors for a variety of possible mental illness issues start in a Recovery Skills Program together. Here, what to expect and what takes place in groups is discussed in detail over five sessions. In this Recovery Skills stage, not all veterans have been as yet diagnosed with PTSD or other ailments but learn the protocols and idiosyncrasies of coming to terms with their illnesses and how treatment can restore us to a better life. During the five week program, one or two Peer Support Specialists assist the facilitator by supporting her/his dialogue and adding our unique perspectives to the new or returning vets.

The second stage is a four week Orientation stage. In this Group, veterans learn in-depth dynamics of therapy; coming to terms and acceptance with their PTSD, as by now, everyone in this Group has been diagnosed or evaluated and are beginning their own regimens of individual therapy. Those with other mental illnesses have been routed to other programs. For the remaining Orientation period these veterans stay together and develop an identity as their own special Group. Again, two Peer Specialists join a staff clinician to offer support and encourage Group members through their future recovery experiences.

I was pleased to be asked to be a peer in Orientation and on the first meeting there were several veterans, new to the system, who had doubts, were anxious, confused and a little frightened.

I happened to start a conversation before Orientation Group with a black guy who expressed concerns over many of the issues that awaited him. We spent awhile talking and he seemed relieved. During Group that evening he was one of the ones to talk the most; about trust, family and meds.

At the end of the session I approached him and praised him for opening up to us.

Then he said something to me that was truly powerful:

"I told you these things because I could tell by your face I could trust you," he said.

And I thought:

"Oh my God!

My face tells people to trust me?"

"I think I believe you."

"Is that what recovery can be?

— One moment; One day;

One Point of Wellness at a time!"

CLOSING

It's been quite a journey getting here. I've learned so much about the person I am and the person I was.

Occasionally, when I'm participating as a peer with veterans of Iraq and Afghanistan or countless other places where returning veterans remind me of myself forty years ago, I'm asked what I might say to encourage them to stay in recovery, and I say:

"Imagine the possibilities.

I'm 63 years old and only realized a short time ago what it means to want to live.

I've mended a strained relationship with my son and together we've discovered how much we have in common. I've realized that who he is has much to do with who I was and who I've become.

I try with all my heart to make sure my daughter doesn't hurt for me. And I thank her for showing me the power of hope and becoming the confident, bright and caring woman she is.

My wife of nearly 40 years sees me smile. She rode with me along every hill and valley of my illness and never wavered — not even once.

She remains to this moment, my steadfast advocate and true love.

Please don't wait like so many of us did.

Seek treatment; Trust treatment; Stay in treatment.

Imagine the possibilities."

RESOURCES FOR VETERANS AND FAMILIES

***Local or County Veterans Service Commisions**
Check your local directories for location and phone number.

***Patient Education Resource Center, Louis Stokes Cleveland VA Medical Center:**
**About Posttraumatic Stress Disorder*
**Understanding Anxiety Disorders*
**The Truth About Anger*

***National Alliance on Mental Illness, www.nami.org**

***Information on VA health care: 1-877-222-8387, www.va.gov/healtheligibility**

***VA benefits line: 1-800-827-1000**

***Department of Veterans Affairs website: www.va.gov**

***The Women's Trauma Treatment Program**
Mental Health Wellness Center
Louis Stokes VA Medical Center
1000 Brecksville Road, Brecksville, Ohio 44141

***Vet Centers:** Free Readjustment Counseling Services for veterans who served during armed hostilities, including family and marital counseling; alcohol/drug assessment; bereavement counseling; sexual trauma counseling and referral services. Vet Centers seem to be especially appealing to state, county and city employees, such as policemen, firemen etc. who are reluctant to reveal personal issues within their departments.

***The Emotional Brain*, book publication, Joseph LeDoux, 1998.**

****Veterans and Families Guide to Recovering from PTSD,*** Stephanie Laite Lanham, PMH-NP, CNS. Published by Purple Heart Service Foundation, PO Box 49, Annandale, VA 22003.
www.purpleheartfoundation.org;
email: phsf@purpleheartfoundation.org.

****Post-Trauma Stress: a personal guide to reduce the long term effects and hidden emotional damage caused by violence and disaster.*** **Frank** Parkinson. 1993, 2000, Da Capo Press, www.dacapopress.com.

****After the War: for the wives of all veterans;*** Pamphlet. **www.patiencepress.com.**